HARDCORE CIRCUIT TRAINING FOR MEN

JIM McHALE

CHOHWORA UDU

PW

PRICE WORLD
PUBLISHING

Prior to beginning any exercise program, you must consult with your physician. You must also consult your physician before increasing the intensity of your training.

Any application of the recommended material in this book is at the sole risk of the reader, and at the reader's discretion. Responsibility of any injuries or other adverse effects resulting from the application of any of the information provided within this book is expressly disclaimed.

Published by Price World Publishing, LLC
1300 W. Belmont Ave, Suite 20G
Chicago, IL 60657

Modeling by Edwin John Yang and Rob Price
Book design and layout by Dianne T. Goh
Interior photographs by Dianne T. Goh
Editing by Sherry Roberts
Printing by Sheridan Books, Inc.

First Edition, January 2010
ISBN: 978-0-9724102-6-7
Library of Congress Control Number: 2009922540

Printed in the United States of America

10 9 8 7 6 5 4 3 2 1

Contents

PART I | Introduction

What is this book?

Bored of the same old gym routines? Lack motivation to get fit? Away from home a lot and can't stick to a training plan? Want to take your fitness training to the next level? Then this book is for you.

Hardcore Circuit Training for Men is a no-nonsense approach to high-intensity fitness training. The exercises and circuits in this book will give you the motivation to get superfit and help you dramatically improve your muscular strength and aerobic fitness.

In a park, a hotel room, a gym with hardly any equipment, or even your living room—there is a circuit here to suit your fitness needs. Now there are no excuses.

Everyone seems to lead busy lives these days, and it can be difficult to find the time or even motivation to fit a workout into a hectic schedule. With that in mind, we have specifically designed these workouts so that you will be able to use at least one of them in most environments in which you find yourself.

Hardcore Circuit Training for Men concentrates on tried-and-tested exercises and equipment, which have all been proven time and again to deliver results.

Who should use this book?

Put simply, anyone interested in getting superfit, specifically:

- Individuals aspiring to lose weight, tone muscle, or get superfit.
- Athletes who want to work on their conditioning.
- Sports teams or team coaches looking for pre-season conditioning inspiration.
- Personal trainers searching for new ideas for their clients.
- Anyone who is bored with his current workouts and wants to try something new.

Who should not use this book?

Anyone with a serious medical condition, especially a heart condition, should seek specific advice from a medical professional before trying any exercises in this book.

Additionally, anyone who has below average physical fitness should consult medical advice before trying the exercises in this book.

Who are the authors of this book?

Jim McHale is an endurance athlete and ex-amateur boxer with more than ten years experience designing gym circuits. He has experience competing in Ironman Triathlon and other long-distance events including the 190 kilometer Libyan Challenge Desert Race. Jim has been associated with the fitness industry for more than 15 years.

Chohwora Udu has more than thirty years experience in boxing as both a professional fighter and as a coach. He has trained both professional and amateur boxers and he holds YMCA qualifications in gym instruction and circuit training. As a fitness instructor, Chohwora specializes in the areas of muscular endurance, strength, and flexibility.

A note on training intensity

The circuits in this book are meant to be hard and intense. If your heart isn't beating fast and you're not sweating, then you're doing something wrong.

If you can afford it, buy a heart rate monitor. This will tell you exactly how hard you are working and help you keep track of which heart rate zone you are working in. The most effective zone for overall cardiovascular fitness is between 70 percent and 80 percent of your working heart rate. Working in this zone generates the best results.

How do I calculate my working heart rate?
Roughly speaking, your maximum heart rate is 220 minus your age.

The formula for your working heart rate is:
Your "maximum heart rate" minus your "resting heart rate" equals your "working heart rate."

Let's look at an example for a twenty-five-year-old athlete:

Maximum heart rate:
220 – 25 = 195 beats per minute (bpm).

Resting heart rate: 55 bpm.

Working heart rate:
195 (maximum heart rate) –55 (resting heart rate)
= 140 bpm (working heart rate)

Now, that we know your working heart rate, we can figure the best zone for training–which is between 70 percent and 80 percent of your working heart rate. This is important because you want to be careful not to go too far over your target zone.

Using the example above, let's calculate your target training zone by adding 80 percent of your working heart rate to your resting heart rate:

140 bpm x 0.8 (80% of working heart rate)
+ 55 (resting heart rate) = 167 bpm (target training zone).

So a twenty-five-year-old athlete with a resting heart rate of 55 beats per minute should be aiming to exercise at around 167 beats per minute.

What this book cannot do for you

There are no magic shortcuts to getting fit. You will have to push your body hard. However, that doesn't mean you need to blindly follow this book without any thought for timing of exercise, nutrition, or rest. Think of exercise as just one of the components you need to get fit.

Remember to train smart–maximize the time you have available for exercise by having a clear idea of what workout you are doing each time you go to the gym.

Ideally, get lots of rest and sleep. Do not train every day; your body needs time to recover after vigorous exercise.

Think about training in pairs or a small group. You will motivate each other, and it helps prevent "cheating" or poor technique during exercises. If you can afford it, exercise with a qualified personal trainer.

Nutrition

Nutrition is a topic all by itself, and we could easily fill a separate book on the subject if we went into any detail. In this book, we are concentrating on exercise so we will only briefly touch on nutrition.

Nutrition is an absolutely essential part of getting fit, but what works for one person may not necessarily work for someone else because we all burn calories at different rates. That said, there are some general rules of thumb to follow:

- Eat little and often. Have several small meals throughout the day whenever you feel hungry rather than a few big meals. Try eating meals around the size of your hand rather than filling the whole plate with food.

- Eat after exercise. If you've just burned a load of calories exercising, then your body will be looking to replace those calories. If you don't eat fairly soon, your body will be likely to start burning muscle to use as fuel, which defeats the whole purpose of exercising in the first place.

- Raw food is better than cooked food. When you cook food, you destroy some of the nutrients inside it. Try eating raw vegetables, fruit, raw fish (sushi), etc. Obviously DON'T eat ALL food raw for health reasons.
- If you want advice and tips on nutrition, take a look at: **www.mensfitness.com/nutrition** and **www.menshealth.co.uk/Nutrition/landing**.

Some Useful Resources

There is a tremendous amount of useful information about exercise and nutrition on the Web. Here is a selection of some of our favorite Web sites:

- **www.dailyburn.com**–Fitness site for detailed tracking of workouts and nutrition, online accountability, and motivation. Free to sign up for an account.
- **www.mensfitness.com**–Web site for monthly fitness magazine featuring good advice on fitness, weight training, and nutrition.
- **www.sportsworkout.com/etraining**–Excellent online personal training site where you can train directly with fitness expert Rob Price.
- **www.mapmyrun.com**–Create/share or search for runs in your area.
- **www.gimme20.com**–Good online resource for creating and finding gym workouts. Offers a volume of details, pictures, and explanations.
- **www.youtube.com**–Search for thousands of fitness videos here; great for picking up tips on technique or for getting new exercise ideas.

Disclaimers, Warnings and Anticipated Questions

The authors and publisher of this book accept no liability for any injury or illness sustained while carrying out the circuits described in this book. You carry out these circuits at your own risk.

Before attempting any of the circuits outlined in this book, please be sure to take some time and learn the proper technique for each exercise. Ideally, this should be with the help of a personal trainer or other physical training professional.

Many of the exercises in this book are not necessarily easy to perform (although most can be modified to match your fitness level). If you have any doubts as to whether you are capable of performing a specific exercise, please consult with your doctor.

Wherever possible, the authors of this book have endeavored to verify the content of third-party Web links and references. However, the authors are not responsible for the content of third-party Web sites and, therefore, cannot be liable for their content. You link to Web sites at your own risk. This book provides Web links and references to you only as a convenience. The inclusion of any link or reference does not imply endorsement by the authors of this book.

Some answers to questions you may want to ask:

"These techniques didn't work for me."

Although these exercises work for most people, we understand they might not work for everyone. If you are not having the success you anticipated, ask yourself these questions:

- Am I training hard enough?
- Am I training too hard?
- Is my technique correct?
- Am I eating correctly?

If in any doubt, contact a personal fitness trainer and ask for some advice.

"You didn't invent these circuits or exercises."

We are not suggesting that we invented these circuits or exercises. In fact, a lot of these exercises have been around for a long time in one form or another. We are just letting you know what has been successful for us.

PART II | The Circuits

Warming Up

The basic idea behind "warming up" is to prepare your body, particularly your muscles, for physical activity.

A warmup is therefore usually performed directly before exercise and involves some kind of low-intensity activity. Jogging is ideal. It increases your heart rate and generally prepares you for what is to come.

Many people include stretching in a warmup, although among fitness professionals, there is some dispute as to what the exact risks and benefits of doing this are. Either way, for our purposes, a form of mild stretching will be fine. It is entirely up to you and how you feel at the time as to what you do.

Take a look at w**ww.netfit.co.uk/stretching.htm** for some stretching examples.

Try to use the following points as a guideline:

- Spend about five minutes warming up.

- Address the areas of your body that you are about to exercise.

- Don't warm up for long periods before explosive exercise.

- Concentrate on any muscles that feel tight. However, if you are injured, don't exercise at all—rest it!

Cooling Down

Warming down or "cooling down" relates to the period straight after exercise where you gradually change from a state of physical exertion to a state of near rest.

Just as with warming up before exercise, it is usually a good idea to warm down after exercise. Warming down has been proven to help remove lactic acid, but as yet, there is no evidence to suggest it reduces muscle soreness after exercise.

Ideally, spend around five minutes jogging, slowly decreasing the intensity as you go. Try to rehydrate yourself during this period or directly afterwards.

As with warming up, stretching can be included as part of a warm down.
Visit **www.netfit.co.uk/stretching.htm**
for some stretching examples.

Body Weight Workout

Our first workout is based entirely on body weight and, therefore, requires no equipment, not even a bench or a step.

It can be completed pretty much anywhere; it doesn't require a lot of room, just enough to be able to lie down on the floor. This makes this workout ideal to use at home, in a hotel, or somewhere indoors. Watch out for clearance above your head on the last exercise, which requires you to perform a jumping jack after the burpee.

DYNAMIC "CLAP" PUSH-UPS

SINGLE ARM PUSH-UPS

"V" CRUNCH SIT-UPS

SIT-UPS

BACK EXTENSIONS

SINGLE-LEG "PISTOL" SQUATS

BURPEES WITH A JUMPING JACK

Equipment Required
No equipment needed.

Instructions
Carry out 4 sets of the 7 exercises.
Take a 1-minute rest between sets.

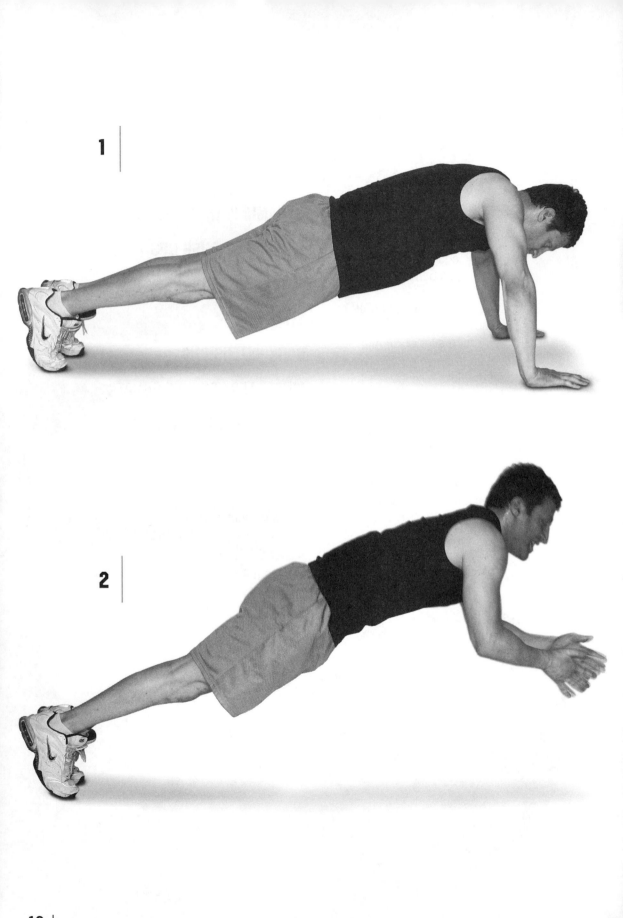

DYNAMIC "CLAP" PUSH-UPS

Reps: 15

Description/Notes:

1 | Hands leave the floor as you push off.

2 | Quickly bring them together (hence "clap") before returning hands to the floor.

For a video of this exercise, visit:

www.youtube.com/watch?v=tiOugruVaGI

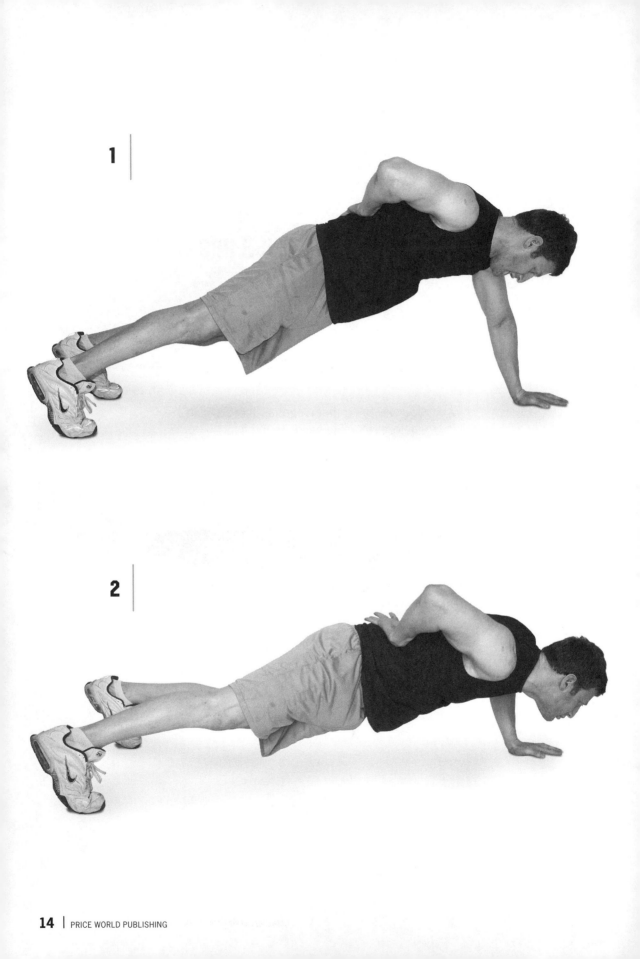

SINGLE ARM PUSH-UPS

Reps: 10 on each arm

Description/Notes:

1 | Keep legs apart for balance.
Position one arm to take your weight and
put your other arm behind your back.

2 | Bend your "working" arm to a
90-degree angle.

For a video of this exercise, visit:

www.youtube.com/watch?v=_fU3KTlth84

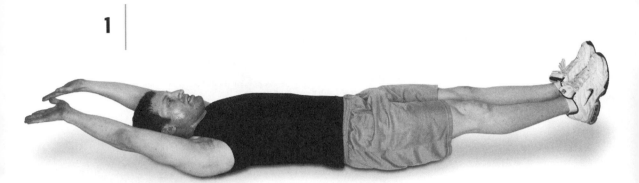

V" CRUNCH SIT-UPS

Reps: 20

Description/Notes:

1 Raise both arms and legs from the lying down "face up" position.

2 Torso should leave the floor. Aim to touch your feet with your hands.

2 |

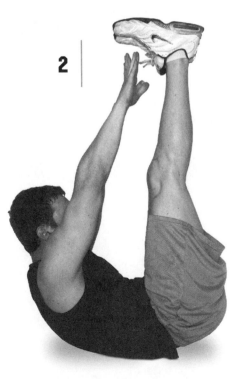

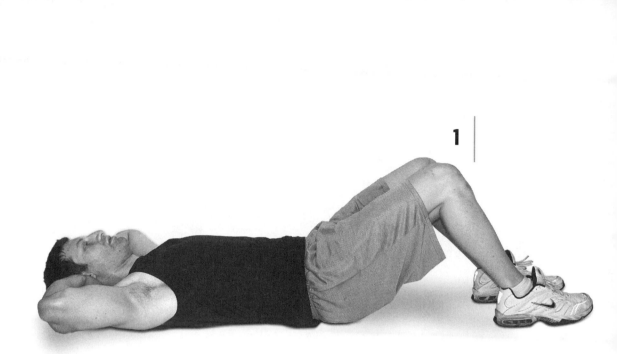

SIT-UPS

Reps: 20

Description/Notes:

1 Keep hands on side of head.

2 Chest should come all the way up to knees.

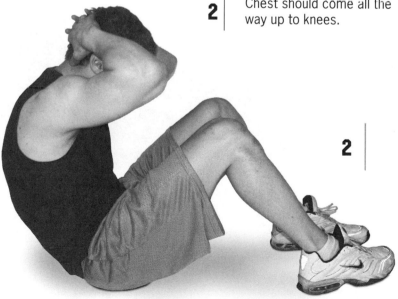

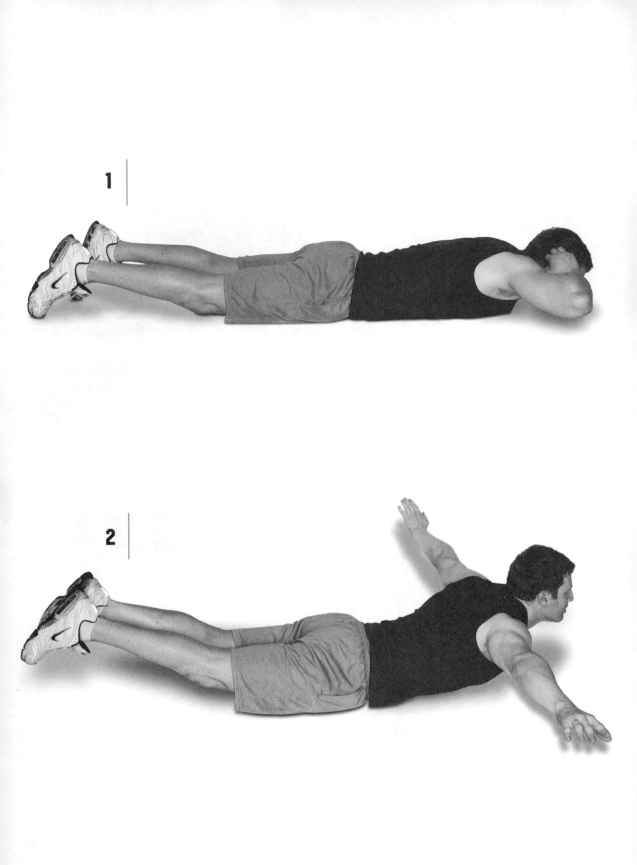

BACK EXTENSIONS

Reps: 20

Description/Notes:

1 | Position yourself lying face down.

2 | Raise both feet and arms off the floor at the same time.

For a video of this exercise, visit:

www.youtube.com/watch?v=iL1cYxmcOSM

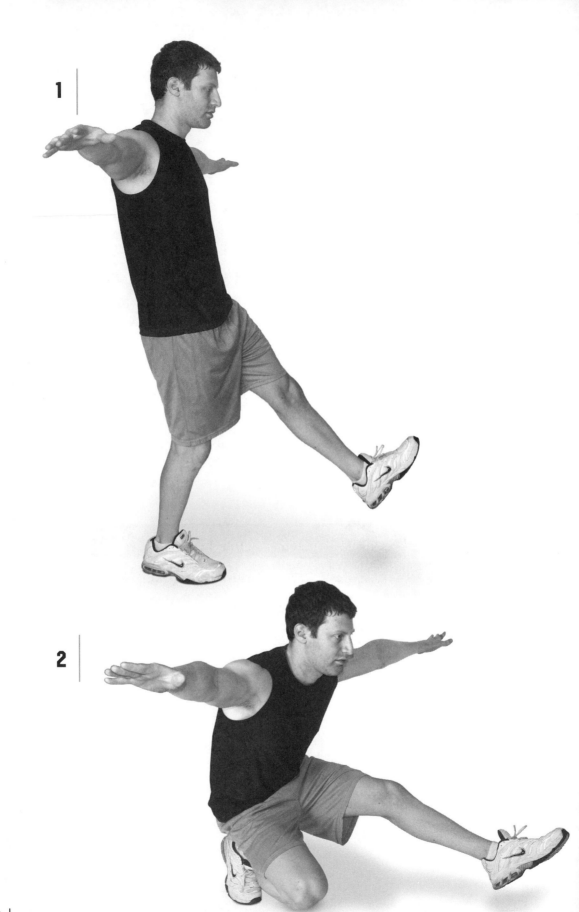

1

2

SINGLE-LEG "PISTOL" SQUATS

Reps: 10 on each leg

Description/Notes:

1 | Balance on one leg with your other leg straight out in front of you.

2 | Bend the leg you are balanced on to 90 degrees, using arms for balance.

For a video of this exercise, visit:

www.youtube.com/watch?v=Hu-6ywxbu1A

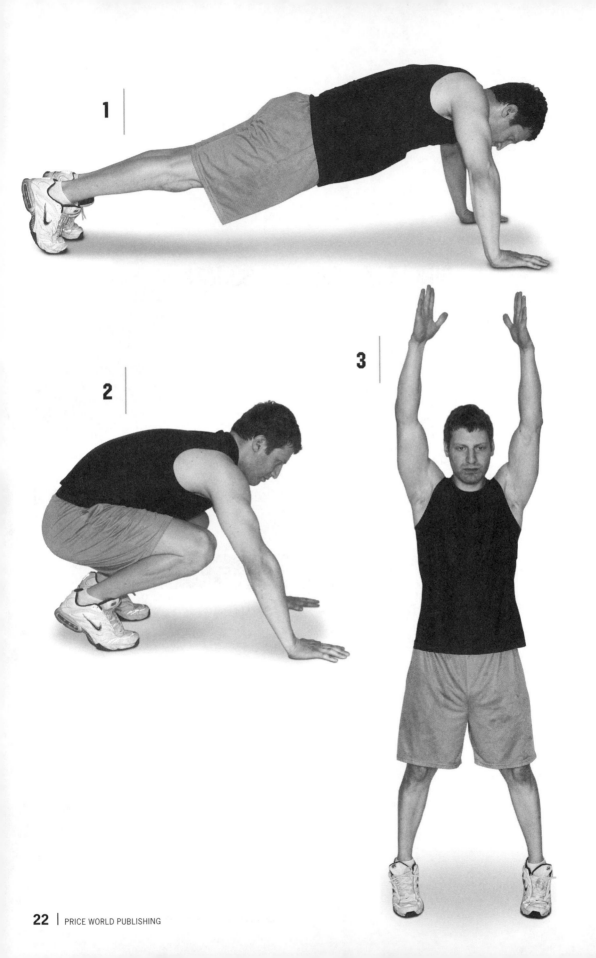

BURPEES WITH A JUMPING JACK

Reps: 20

Description/Notes:

1	To perform a burpee, start in the push-up position.
2	Bring your knees to your chest.
3	Then stand up performing a jumping jack before returning to your original position.

For a video of this exercise, visit:

www.youtube.com/watch?v=c_Dq_NCzj8M

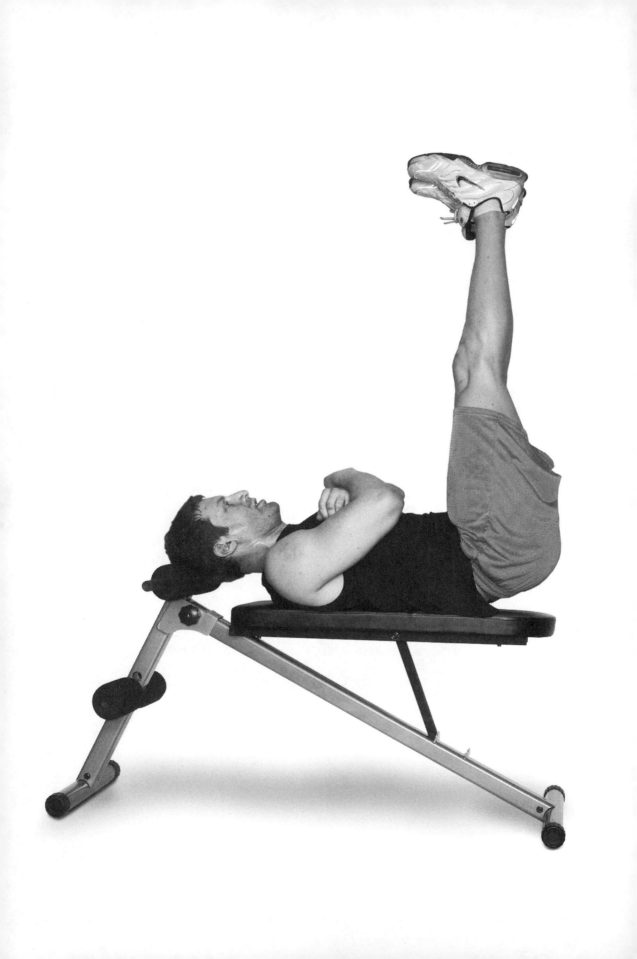

The Bench Workout

As the name suggests, all you need to carry out this workout is a bench or step, so it's ideal for indoors, outdoors, or anywhere you don't have access to much equipment.

Anyone tempted to "cheat" and go for a bench low to the floor will be in for a nasty surprise on the last exercise. So stick with a bench measuring around twenty-four inches off the floor

INCLINED DYNAMIC PUSH-UPS—ON AND OFF BENCH

"SPIDERMAN" PUSH-UPS WITH FEET ON BENCH

"V" CRUNCHES—LEGS OFF THE BENCH

LEG RAISES

TRICEP DIPS—LEGS STRAIGHT

BOX JUMPS

SINGLE-LEG "PISTOL" SQUATS FROM SITTING POSITION

Equipment Required

A bench or equivalent–roughly 24 inches above the floor.

Instructions

Carry out 4 sets of the 7 exercises.
Take a 1-minute rest between sets.

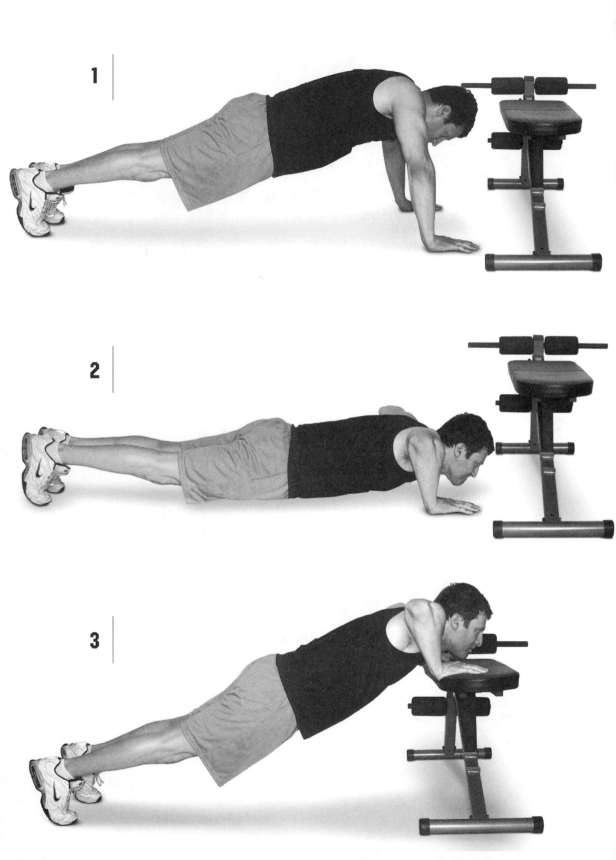

1

2

3

INCLINED DYNAMIC PUSH-UPS–
ON AND OFF BENCH

Reps: 20

Description/Notes:

1	Start in the push-up position on the floor with your head near the bench.
2	Push off the floor with your hands explosively.
3	Both hands should leave the floor and finish up on the bench. Get back in the push-up position on the floor to start the exercise over again.

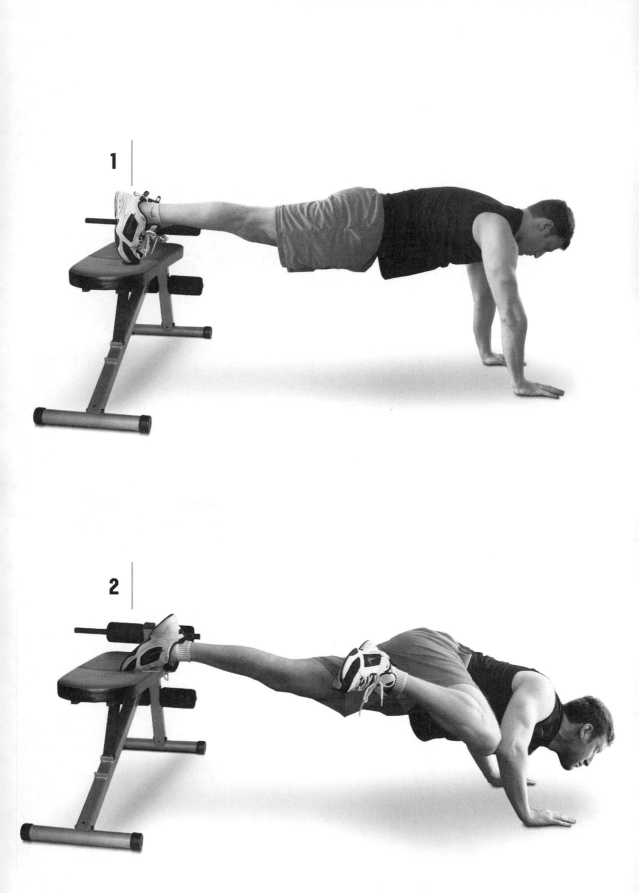

"SPIDERMAN" PUSH-UPS
WITH FEET ON BENCH

Reps: 15

Description/Notes:

1 | Start with your feet on the bench and hands on the floor in the push-up position.

2 | As you press down, bring alternate knees to your elbows.

For a video of this exercise, visit:

www.youtube.com/watch?v=eHbJoeA1I4E

1

"V" CRUNCHES–
LEGS OFF THE BENCH

Reps: 30

Description/Notes:

1 | Lie on the bench, face up.

2 | Raise both arms and legs from the lying face-up position. Torso should leave the bench. Aim to touch your feet with your hands.

2

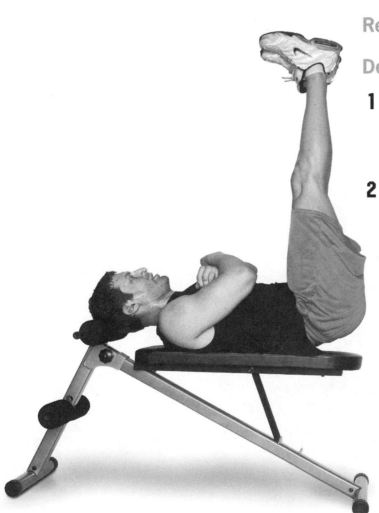

LEG RAISES

Reps: 30

Description/Notes:

1 Lie on the bench, face up with your legs off the bench and both legs together.

2 Keeping both legs together, raise legs to 90 degrees then lower in a controlled manner back to the original position. Keep torso flat on the bench.

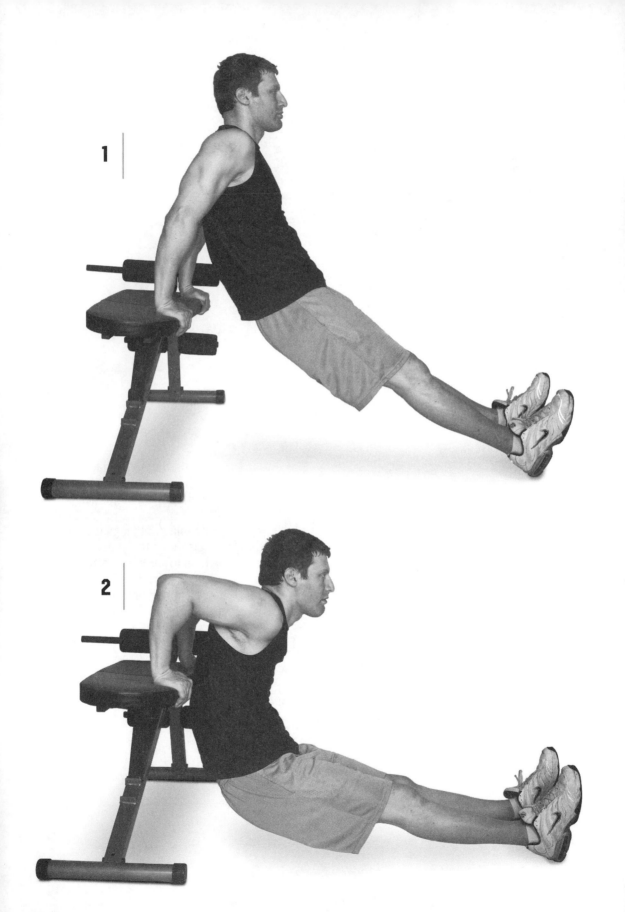

TRICEP DIPS-LEGS STRAIGHT

Reps: 30

Description/Notes:

1
Start with both hands on the bench and arms straight supporting your weight. Stretch legs out in front of you, feet on the floor. Legs should be only slightly bent at the knee.

2
Lower your body by bending your elbows slowly until they are bent 90 degrees. Then slowly straighten your arms until you are back in the start position.

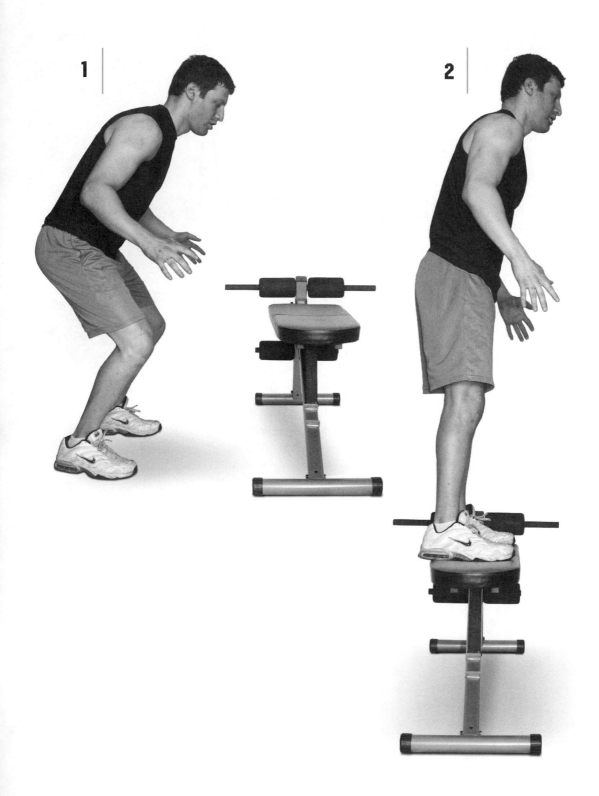

BOX JUMPS

Reps: 30

Description/Notes:

1 | Stand facing the bench.

2 | Jump (using both legs, keeping them together) onto the bench and then back onto the floor. Do not step onto the bench.

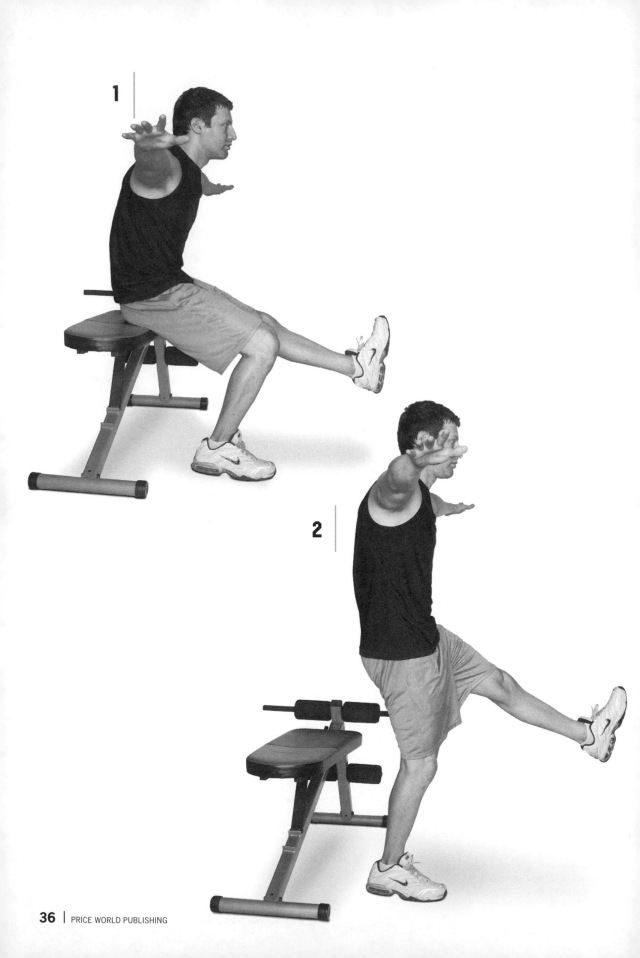

1

2

SINGLE-LEG "PISTOL" SQUATS FROM SITTING POSITION

Reps: 10 on each leg

Description/Notes:

1	Sit down on the bench, only one foot on the floor. Stand up using only one leg and suspending the other leg off the floor.
2	Slowly sit down and repeat.

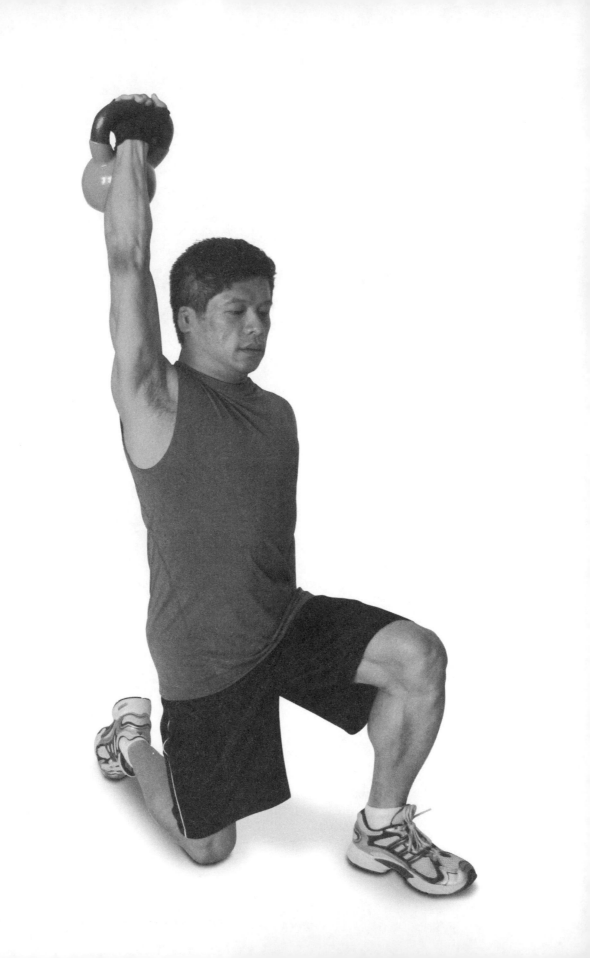

Kettlebell Workout

Kettlebells are a type of weight used specifically for strength and fitness training. If you haven't come across them before, please take a look at this Web site for a full description: **www.en.wikipedia.org/ wiki/Kettlebell**. In recent years, they have become more popular, thanks in part to their use among professional athletes. You should be able to find kettlebells in most well-stocked gyms. If you can't find them, don't worry about it. For the purposes of this circuit, dumbbells can be substituted for kettlebells and should work just as well.

PUSH-UPS OFF KETTLEBELL INTO SINGLE-ARM ROWS

SINGLE-ARM BENCH PRESSES

SINGLE-HAND KETTLEBELL CLEAN AND PRESS

KETTLEBELL SWINGS

TURKISH "GET-UPS"

RUSSIAN TWISTS– LEGS RAISED OFF THE FLOOR

FULL SIT-UP WITH KETTLEBELL

Equipment Required

Two sets of kettlebells (weight loads depend upon your ability and size)

Instructions

Carry out 4 sets of the 7 exercises

Take a 1-minute rest between sets.

1

PUSH-UPS OFF KETTLEBELL INTO SINGLE-ARM ROWS

Reps: 20

Description/Notes:

1 Start this exercise in the push-up position with each hand on a kettlebell handle.

2 Perform a full push-up then, staying in the push-up position, lift each kettlebell your chest, one after the other.
This is 1 repetition.

2

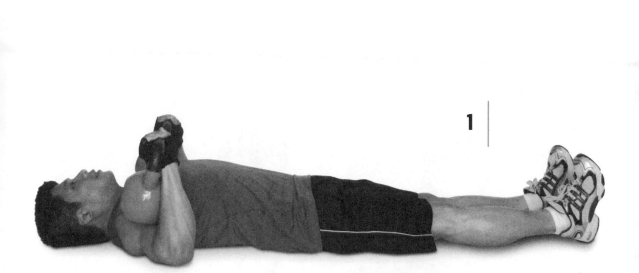

SINGLE-ARM BENCH PRESSES

Reps: 10 on each arm

Description/Notes:

1 | Lie on the floor facing up. Hold a kettlebell in each hand.

2 | One at a time, press each kettlebell vertically until your arm is almost straight. Then return it to the starting position.

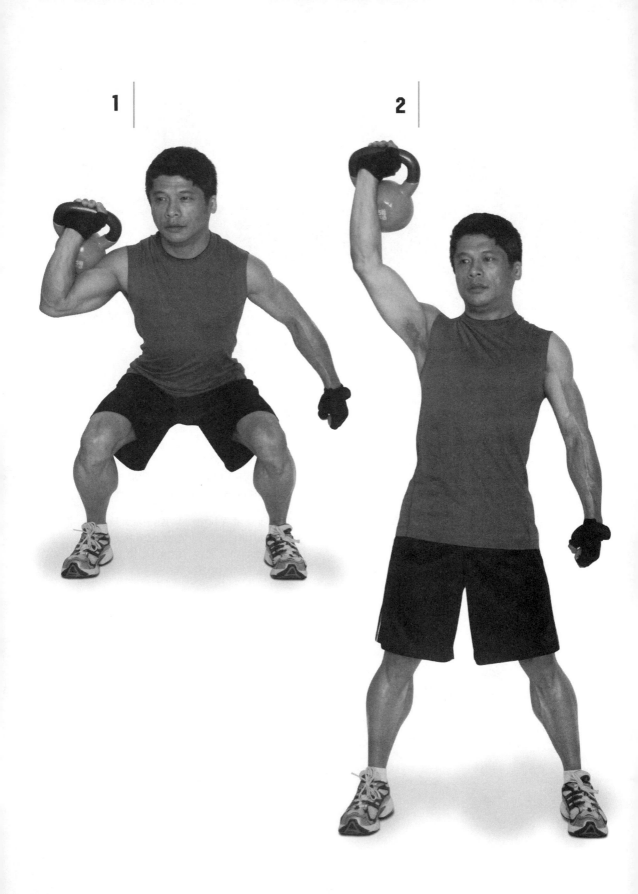

SINGLE-HAND KETTLEBELL CLEAN AND PRESS

Reps: 10 on each arm

Description/Notes:

1 | Position the kettlebell between your legs, back straight, knees bent.

2 | Clean the kettlebell in one dynamic motion, and then press it above your head.

To perform a kettlebell clean, pull the kettlebell up explosively, and when it reaches your mid thighs, shrug it up while simultaneously dropping yourself beneath it and performing what is effectively a reverse curl.

For a video of this exercise, visit:

www.youtube.com/watch?v=-T3FH3VNILo

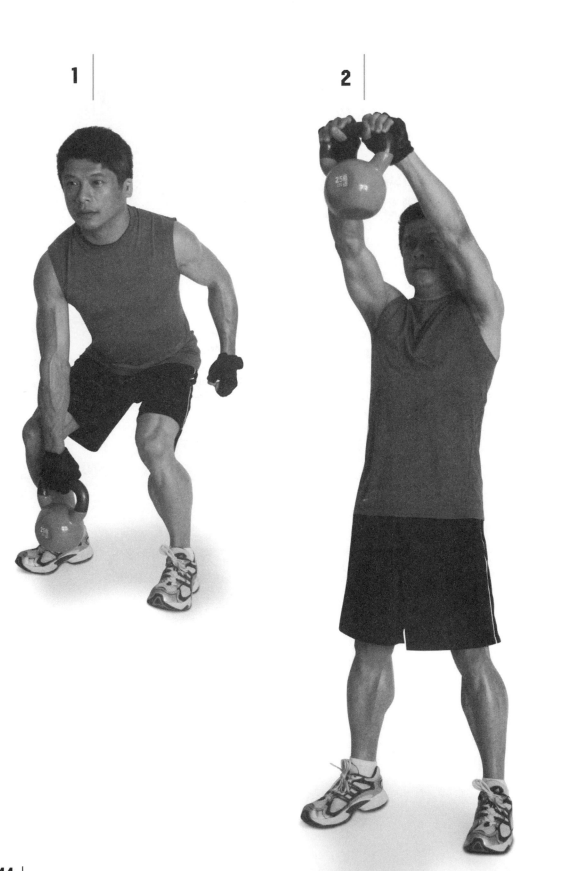

1

2

KETTLEBELL SWINGS

Reps: 10 on each arm

Description/Notes:

1 | Stand with your back straight and knees bent.

2 | Swing kettlebell from between legs up to in line with your head. Change hands at the top of the swing.

For a video of this exercise, visit:

www.youtube.com/watch?v=W1UVCto6xMQ

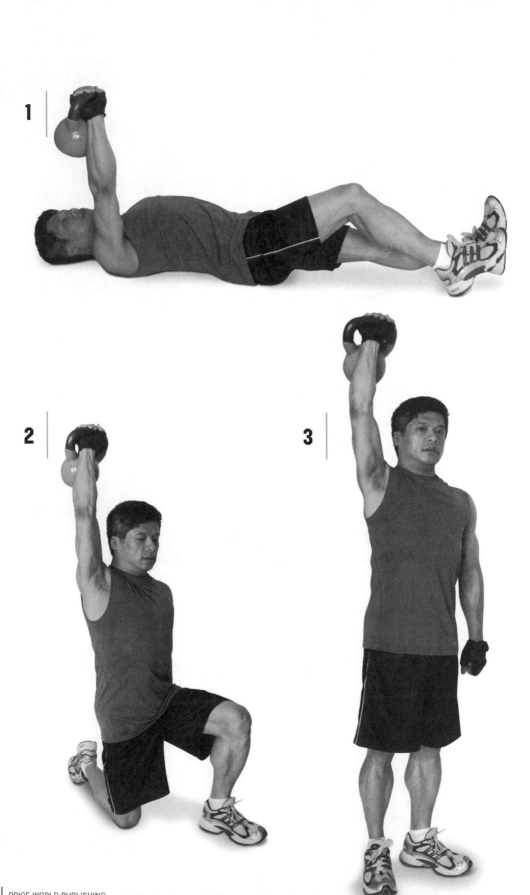

TURKISH "GET-UPS"

Reps: 6 on each side

Description/Notes:

1 Lie face up on the floor with your right knee bent and a kettlebell in your right hand close to your chest. Extend your arm up and away from your body. With the kettlebell still extended above your head, sit up.

2 Using your left hand for support, lift your hips off the ground and bring your left leg through to adopt a lunge position.

3 With the kettlebell still extended above your head, stand up, keeping your legs shoulder-width apart. Return to the starting position using the same technique in reverse.

Once you have completed 6 repetitions, repeat with your other arm.

There a number of variations of this exercise. For examples, check out the following URL:

http://www.youtube.com/watch?v=ztTOnOrSMis

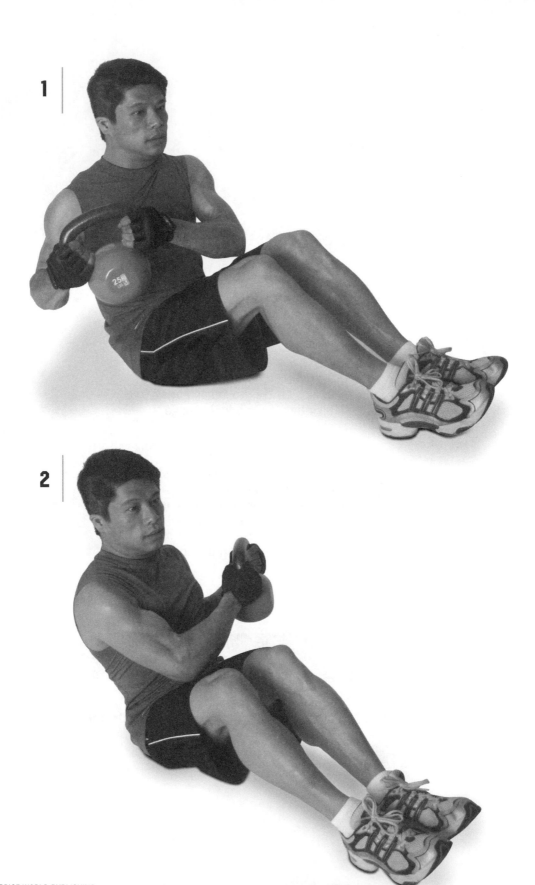

RUSSIAN TWISTS-LEGS RAISED OFF THE FLOOR

Reps: 40

Description/Notes:

1 Start by sitting on the floor with your legs spread out in front of you. Hold the kettlebell to your chest then raise your legs off the floor, bending your knees. At this point you are basically balancing in a "V" position. Once in this balanced position and still gripping the kettlebell with both hands, twist your torso to one side and lower the kettlebell to just off the floor.

2 Then return to the starting position and perform the twist on the other side of your body. This counts as one repetition.

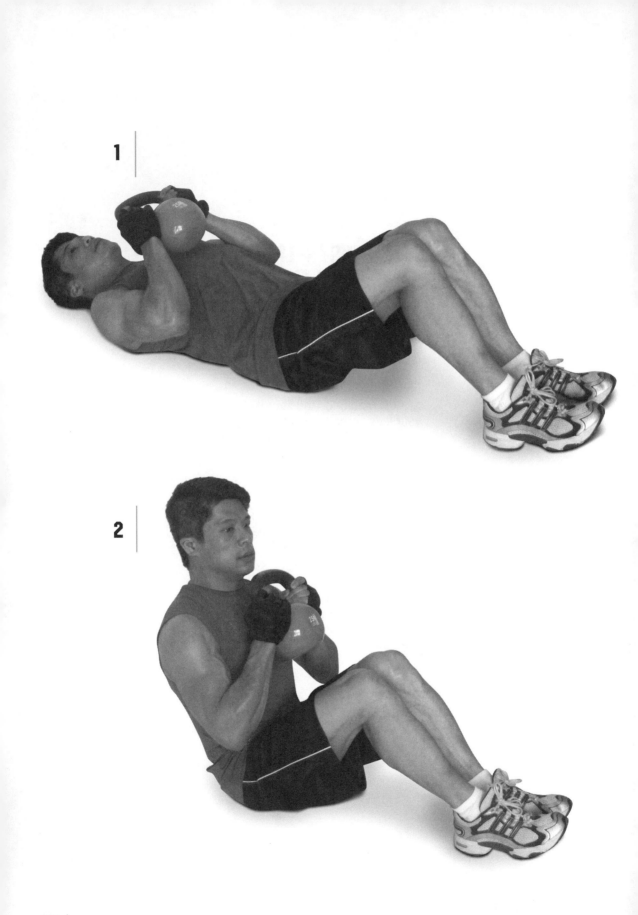

1

2

FULL SIT-UP WITH KETTLEBELL

Reps: 30

Description/Notes:

1 | Start by sitting on the floor, legs out in front of you with knees bent and feet on the floor. Hold the kettlebell close to your chest with both hands.

2 | As with a "normal" sit-up, lower your torso and head to the floor, then sit up keeping the kettlebell to your chest.

If you have problems keeping your feet on the floor, try wedging them under a bar or equivalent.

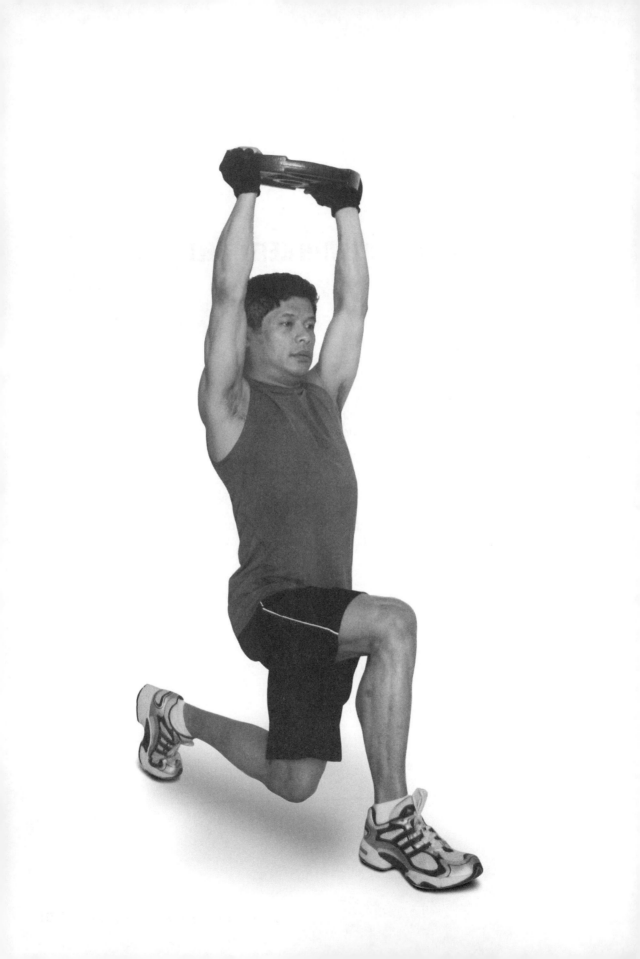

Plate Workout

Common to most gyms are the plates used to stack barbells. In busy gyms, there may be a line to use barbells or dumbbells, but generally you will always find a spare plate lying around to carry out this circuit.

It also requires little space to perform, so it is suitable to do at home or in a hotel room. Feel free to substitute a dumbbell for the plate. If you are really stuck, use a rock or something else heavy enough to give you a good workout.

2 PHASE ARM/SHOULDER PRESS

PLATE ARM FLY

PIKE SIT-UP WITH PLATE

EXTENDED ABDOMINAL CRUNCH WITH PLATE

DYNAMIC SCISSOR LUNGES

PLATE SQUAT

OVERHEAD FORWARD LUNGES

Equipment Required

One plate (weight load depends upon your ability and size).

Instructions

Carry out 4 sets of the 7 exercises.

Take a 1-minute rest between sets.

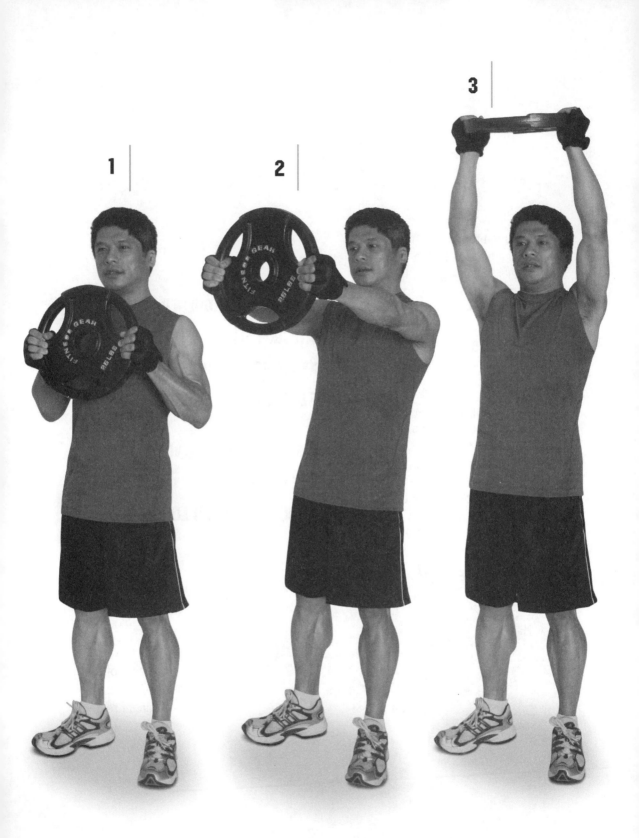

1

2

3

2 PHASE ARM/ SHOULDER PRESS

Reps: 25

Description/Notes:

1 Stand upright with feet shoulder-width apart. Hold the plate close to your chest with both hands.

2 Phase 1: Push the plate out 90 degrees from your body then back to your chest.

3 Phase 2: Push the plate above your head then back down to your chest. This is 1 repetition.

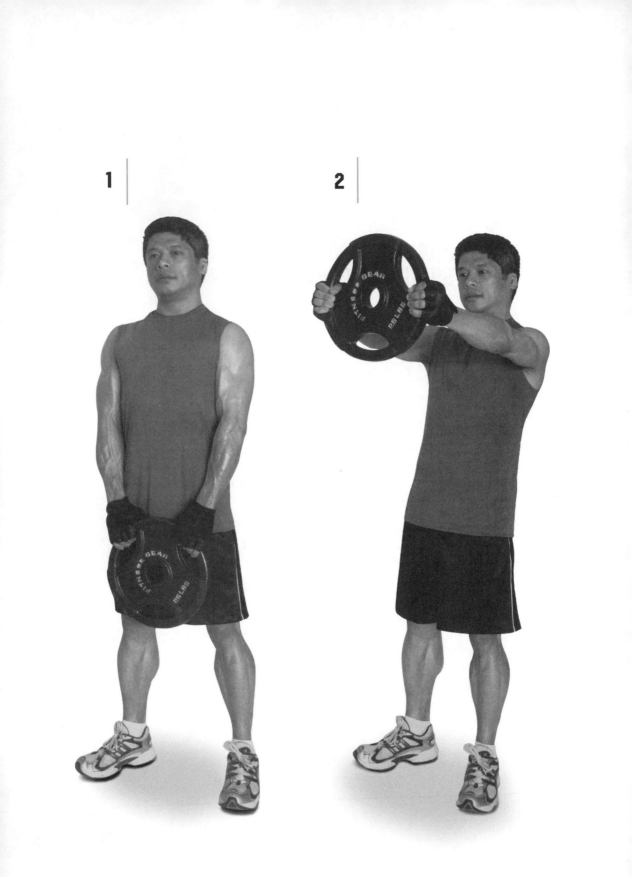

PLATE ARM FLY

Reps: 20

Description/Notes:

1 | Stand upright with feet shoulder-width apart. Hold the plate with straight arms down in front of you.

2 | Lift the plate with straight arms to 90 degrees, perpendicular to your body. Do this in a controlled manner.

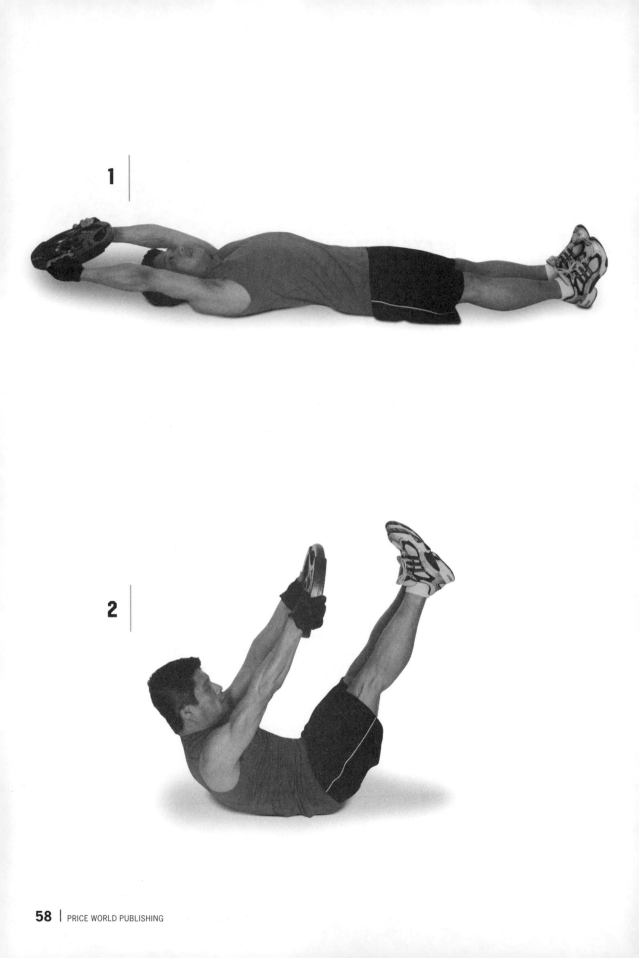

PIKE SIT-UP WITH PLATE

Reps: 20

Description/Notes:

1 Lie face up on the floor with legs flat on the floor and arms stretched above your head, holding the plate. At the same time, lift your legs and arms (keeping them straight) into the pike position–i.e., 90 degrees to the floor.

2 Your feet should touch the plate, and then both feet and arms should return to the floor in a controlled manner.

For a video of this exercise, visit:

www.youtube.com/watch?v=sTYdRiLfuOO

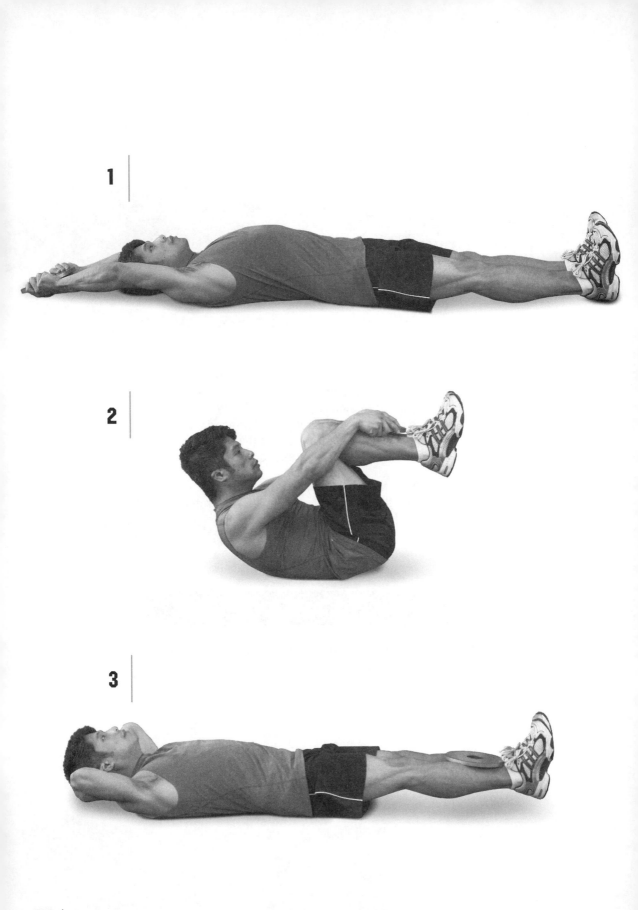

1

2

3

EXTENDED ABDOMINAL CRUNCH WITH PLATE

Reps: 20

Description/Notes:

1 Lie face up on the floor with legs flat on the floor and arms stretched above your head, holding the plate.

2 Perform a "crunch" by bringing your knees into your chest, placing the plate on your shins.

3 Extend your legs back out so they are straight. Then bring your knees back into your chest, take hold of the plate with your hands, and return to the start position. This counts as 1 repetition.

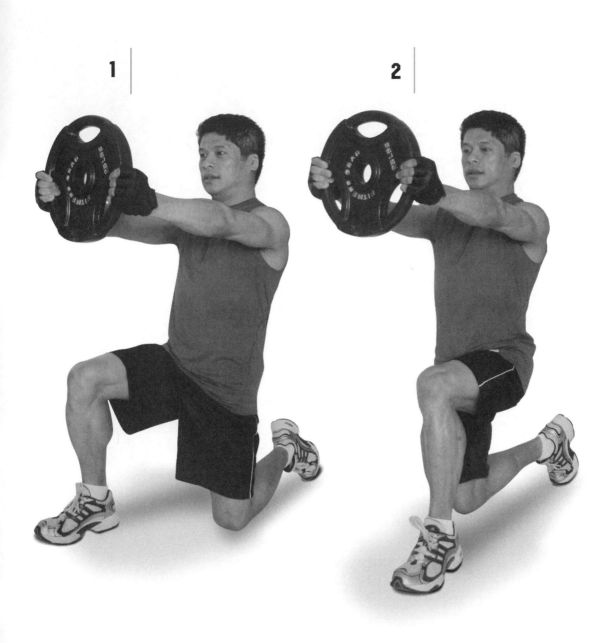

DYNAMIC SCISSOR LUNGES

Reps: 20

Description/Notes:

1 Start in the lunge position, standing with right leg stretched out in front of you, bent at the knee. The left leg should be straight out behind you. Hold the plate with straight arms out in front of you at 90 degrees to your body.

2 Dynamically jump and reverse your leg positions keeping your torso in an upright position. Do this again so your right leg returns to its original position, in front of you. This is 1 repetition.

For a video of this exercise, visit:

www.youtube.com/watch?v=1kBYCMFIjLM

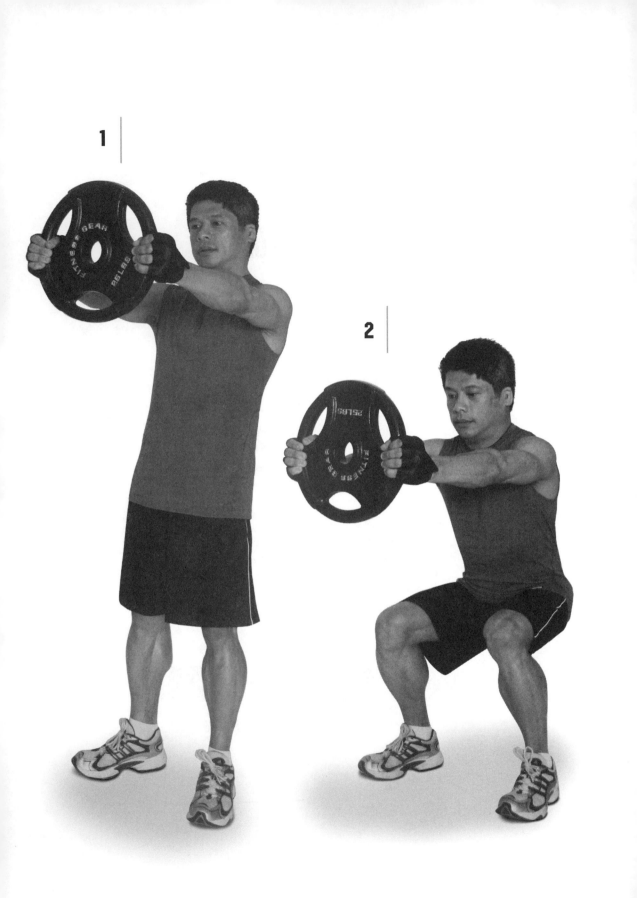

PLATE SQUAT

Reps: 20

Description/Notes:

1 | Stand upright with feet shoulder-width apart. Hold the plate in front of you at 90 degrees, arms straight.

2 | Perform a deep squat so you are in a sitting position, then slowly "stand up" so you return to the starting position.

For a video of this exercise, visit:

www.youtube.com/watch?v=Xmlqihg4VKE

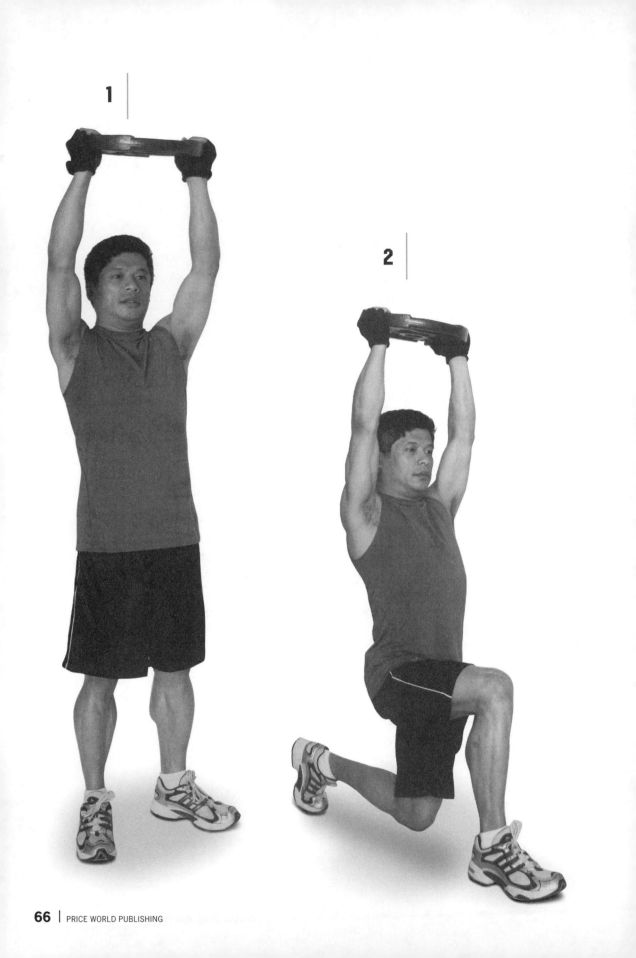

OVERHEAD FORWARD LUNGES

Reps: 20

Description/Notes:

1 Stand upright with feet shoulder-width apart. Hold the plate above your head with straight arms.

2 Take a big step forward with your right leg until your right knee is at a 90-degree angle. Be careful not to lean forward or transfer too much weight to your right leg. Then step back to your original position and rcpeat with your left leg.
This is 1 repetition.

For a video of this exercise, visit:

www.youtube.com/watch?v=p9tS6ErECUo

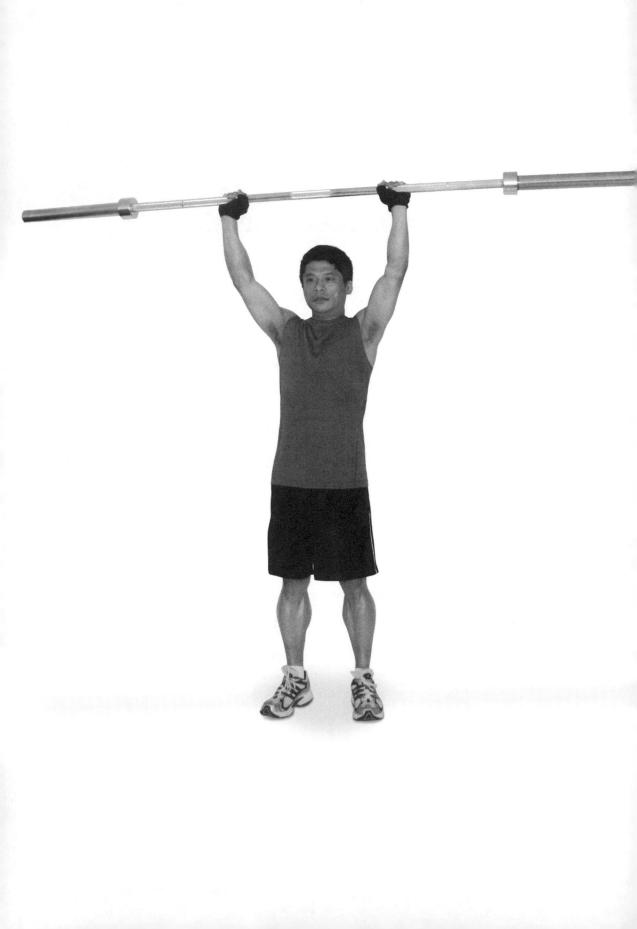

Barbell Workout

The following workout is based on a high-intensity weight training circuit used by Ultimate Fighting Championship and mixed martial arts legend, Randy Couture (www.en.wikipedia.org/wiki/Randy_Couture), as part of his conditioning training.

As Randy says in the youtube.com video where he demonstrates the circuit (**www.youtube.com/watch?v=ArrnEsyaJj4**), the goal is not to "bulk up" but to improve muscle endurance and stamina. During the first or second sets, you may be tempted to think that the circuit is too easy, but by the fifth set, you will have changed your mind. If it's good enough for a five-time UFC champion, it's good enough for you.

The workout does not require a great deal of room and could easily be carried out at home or in a small garden. One thing to watch out for is clearance above your head as two of the exercises require you to shoulder press the barbell.

BENT OVER UPRIGHT ROW

UPRIGHT ROW

SHOULDER PRESS
(BARBELL IN FRONT OF FACE)

SQUATS (LEGS CLOSE TOGETHER)

LUNGES

HANG CLEANS

Equipment Required

One barbell; two plates (weight load depends upon your ability and size).

Instructions

Carry out 5 sets of the 7 exercises.

Take a 1-minute rest between sets.

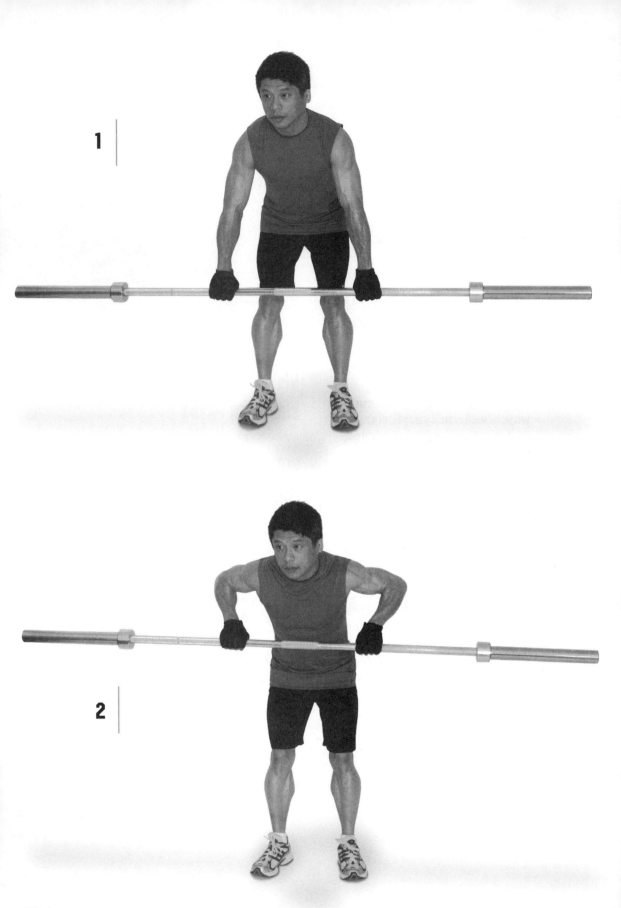

1

2

BENT OVER UPRIGHT ROW

Reps: 8

Description/Notes:

1 | Start in a standing position holding the bar with straight arms and an overhand grip down in front of you.

2 | With knees slightly bent, lean your body over slightly. Bring the bar up to your midriff then slowly back down.

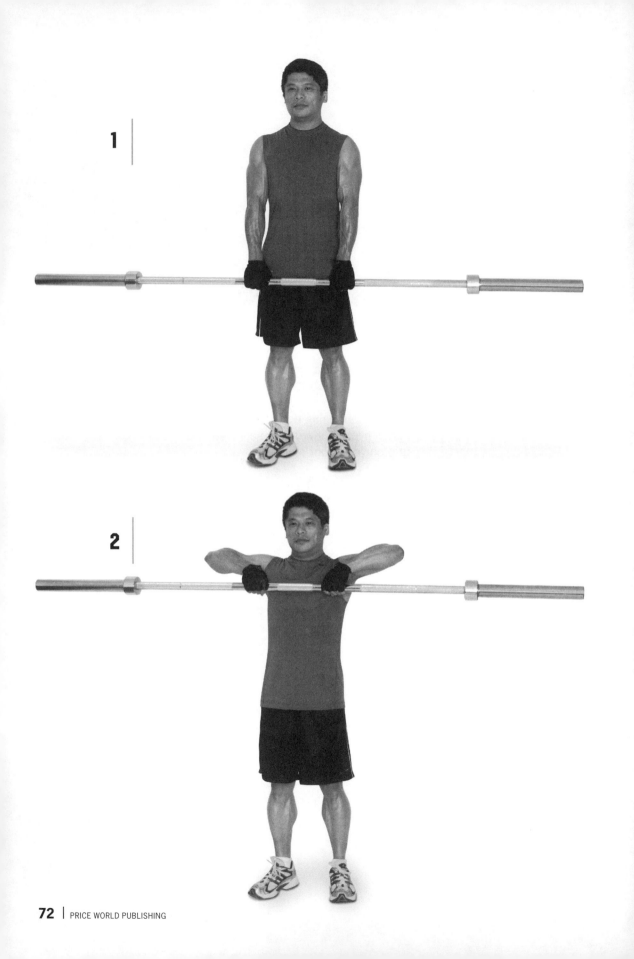

UPRIGHT ROW

Reps: 8

Description/Notes:

| 1 | Start in a standing position holding the bar with straight arms and an overhand grip down in front of you. Back and legs straight. |
| 2 | Bring the bar up to your chest and then slowly back down to the starting position. |

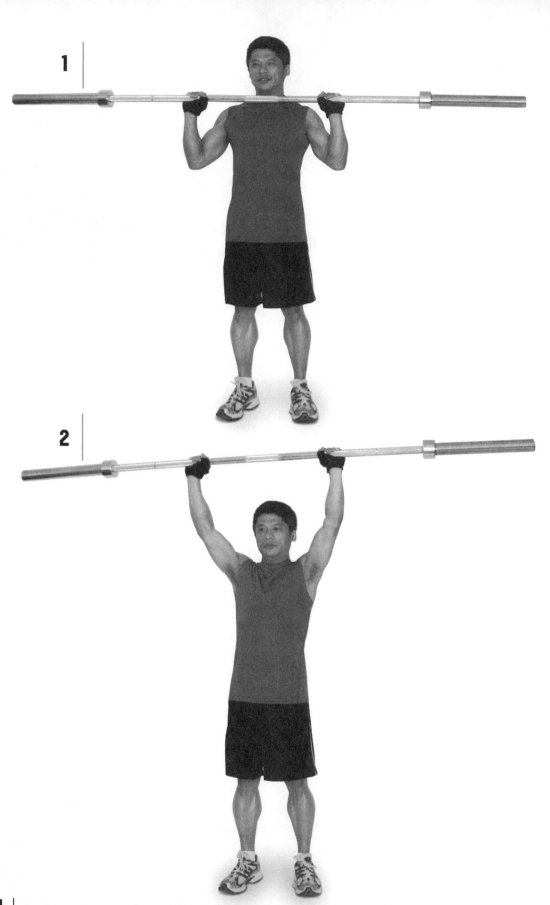

SHOULDER PRESS
(BARBELL IN FRONT OF FACE)

Reps: 8

Description/Notes:

1 | Standing up, hold the bar with an overhand grip. Start with the bar positioned just above your chest, arms bent.

2 | Press the bar above your head, making sure your arms are extended, then return the bar back down to your chest under control.

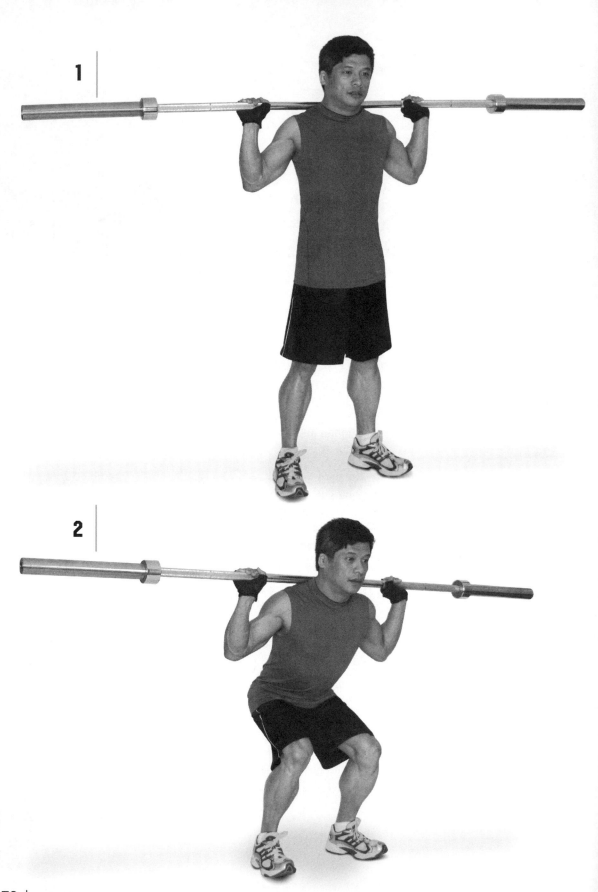

1

2

SQUATS
(LEGS CLOSE TOGETHER)

Reps: 8

Description/Notes:

1 | Position the bar on your shoulders (use some padding on the bar if necessary).

2 | Keeping your legs reasonably close together, bend your knees–keep your back straight as if you are sitting down on a chair. When your knee joint is at 90 degrees, push up into the upright starting position.

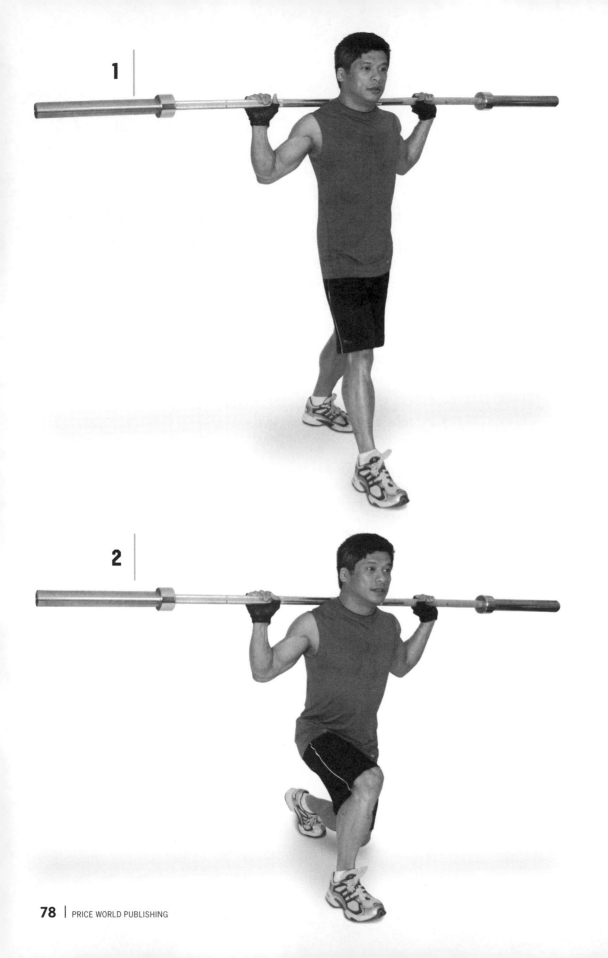

LUNGES

Reps: 16 (8 each leg)

Description/Notes:

1   Start in the lunge position–i.e.,
    as if you were taking a big stride.
    Bar should be on your shoulders.
    Hold it with both hands to balance.

2   Then bend the knee in front of you to
    90 degrees making sure your weight
    is evenly distributed. Return slowly to
    start position. Once 8 repetitions are
    complete, switch legs.

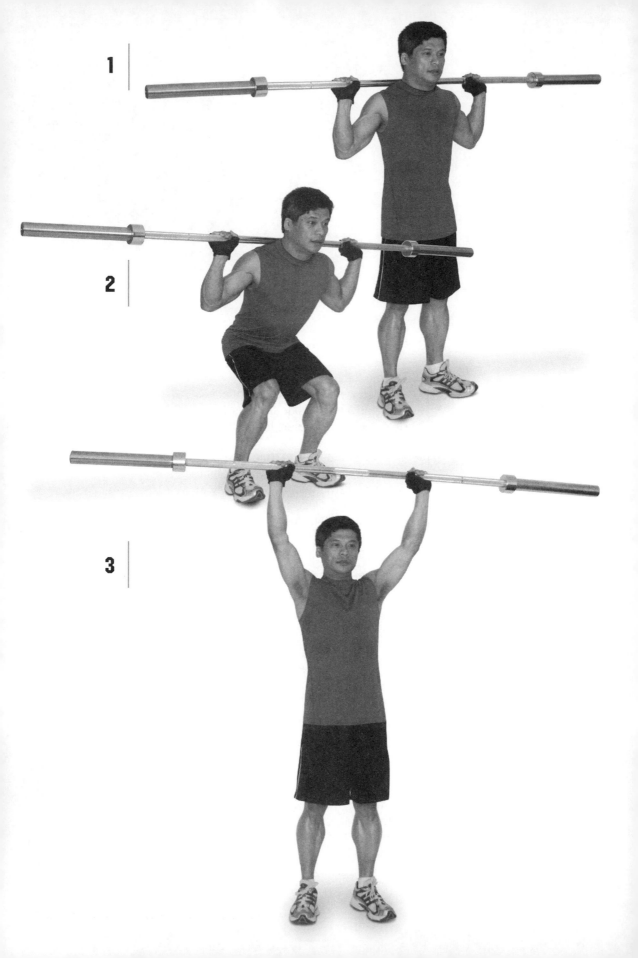

DEEP SQUAT WITH
SHOULDER PRESS
(BARBELL BEHIND HEAD)

Reps: 8

Description/Notes:

1 | Position the bar on your shoulders.

2 | Perform a deep squat (knees bent to 90 degrees), and return to upright position.

3 | Press the bar above your head, returning it to behind your head under control. This is 1 repetition.

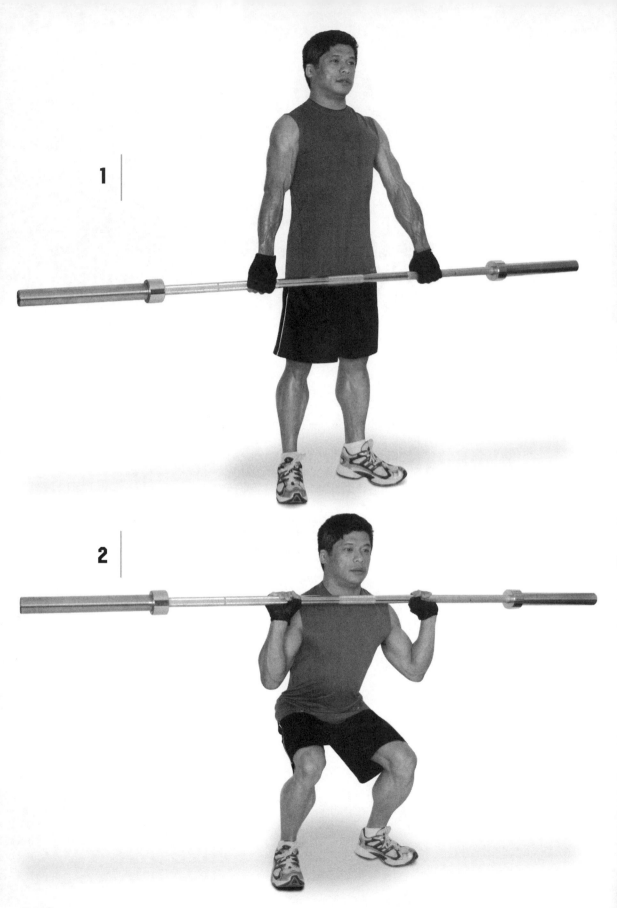

1

2

HANG CLEANS

Reps: 8

Description/Notes:

1 | Stand holding the barbell down in front of you, with an overhand grip slightly wider than shoulder width. Shrug your shoulders and pull the barbell upward with your arms.

2 | Catch the bar on your shoulders while moving into a squat position. Once you hit the bottom of the squat, stand up immediately.

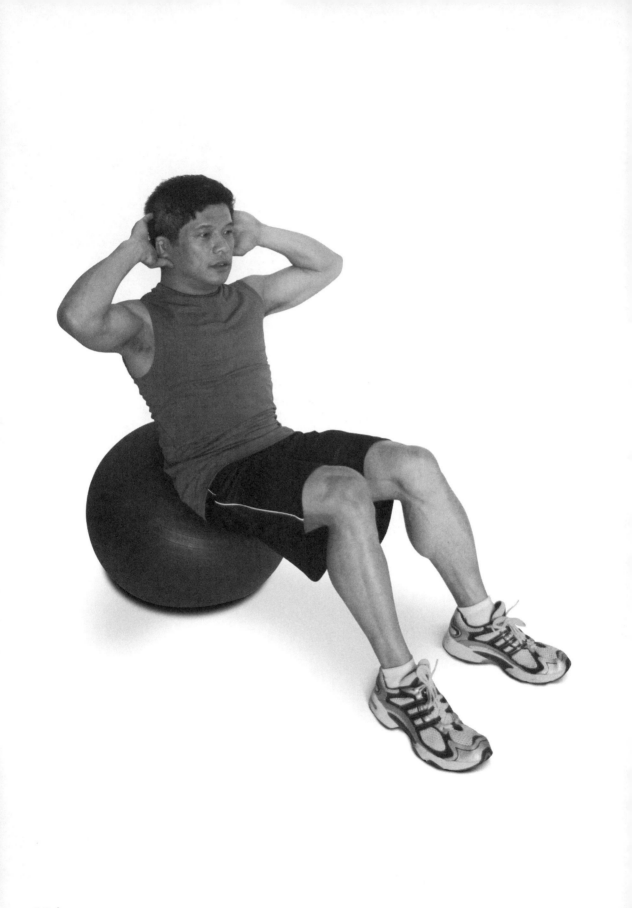

Swiss Ball Workout

Contrary to what some might think, Swiss balls are not just for the delicate and feeble. Just ask Frank Shamrock (**www.youtube.com/watch?v=C_jz-t6_GBg**). The Swiss ball or stability ball (www.en.wikipedia.org/wiki/Swiss_ball) can be found in most gyms. Originally used for clinical physiotherapy, it is now widely used by athletes and personal trainers.

The main benefit of using the ball for exercise is that your body responds to the instability of the ball and engages more muscles to keep you balanced. It is therefore ideal for improving your core strength and balance.

Be careful with this workout. Some of the exercises are advanced and should not be attempted unless you have used a Swiss ball before. If in doubt, you can modify some of the harder exercises to make them a bit easier.

PUSH-UPS
(HANDS ON SWISS BALL)

JACKKNIFE PIKE
(FEET ON SWISS BALL)

SWISS BALL SQUAT
(AGAINST WALL)

SWISS BALL "PLANK"
(FEET ON SWISS BALL)

SWISS BALL CRUNCH
(LIE ON BALL)

SWISS BALL HAMSTRING CURL

REVERSE WOODCHOPS KNEELING ON SWISS BALL

Equipment Required

One Swiss ball (size of Swiss ball should be varied according to your size); one dumbbell (weight load depends upon your ability and size).

Instructions

Carry out 4 sets of the 7 exercises.

Take a 1-minute rest between sets.

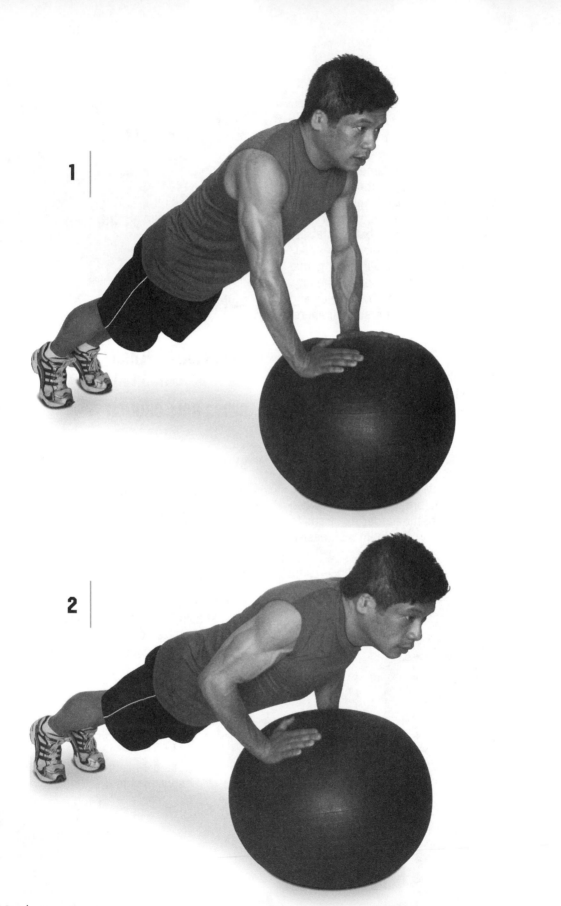

PUSH-UPS
(HANDS ON SWISS BALL)

Reps: 20

Description/Notes:

1 | Place the ball on the floor and position your hands on the ball so you are in full control of it. Assume the push-up position, feet on the floor and hands on the ball.

2 | Maintaining full control, perform a push-up by lowering your chest to the ball, keeping back straight.

For a video of this exercise, visit:

www.youtube.com/watch?v=r6e8DCFTwj4

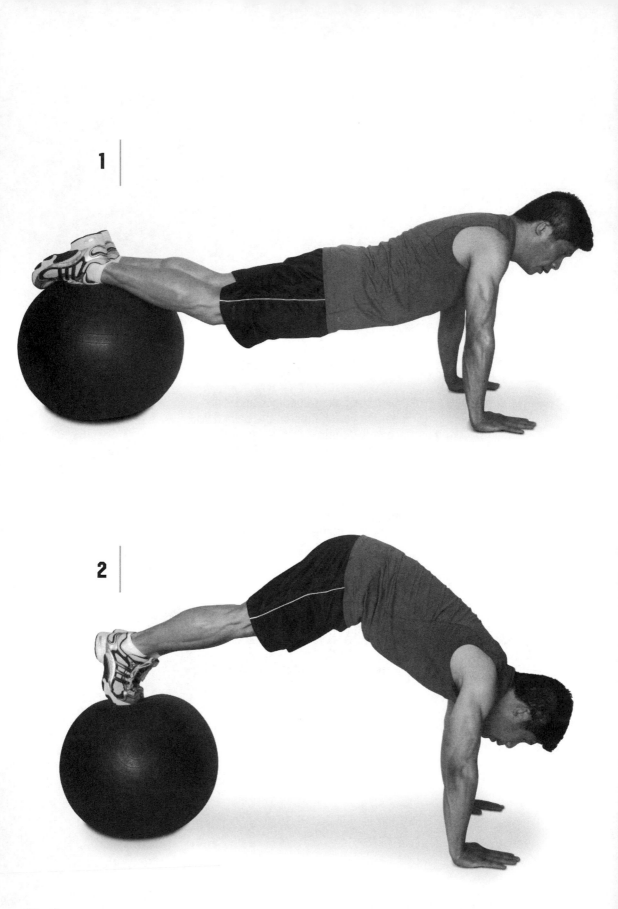

JACKKNIFE PIKE
(FEET ON SWISS BALL)

Reps: 20

Description/Notes:

1 | Assume the push-up position with your feet balanced on top of the ball.

2 | Roll the ball toward you using your feet while keeping your legs straight. Naturally you will assume the pike position—which is torso at 90 degrees to the floor and body bent at the waist, legs straight. Roll the ball back to the start position to complete the exercise.

For a video of this exercise, visit:

www.youtube.com/watch?v=Plx4JGxwL8c

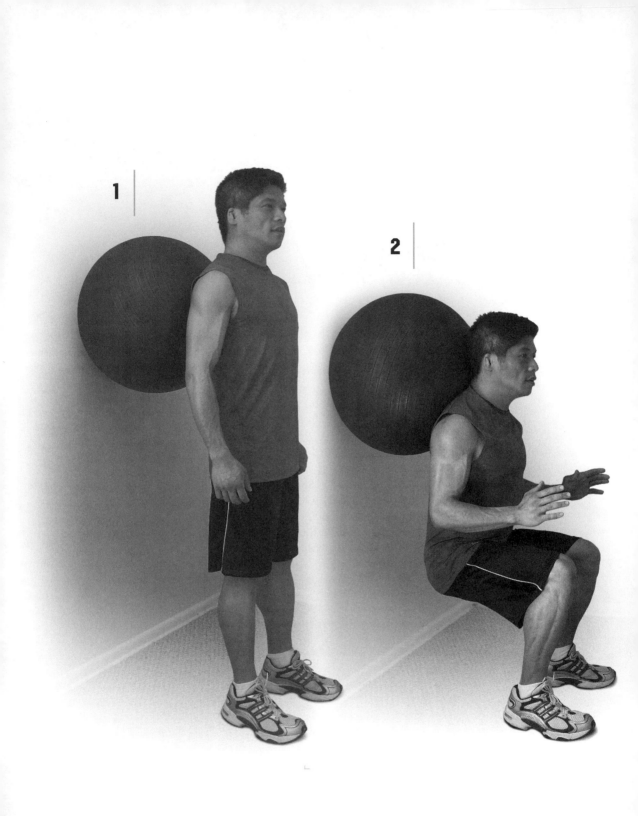

SWISS BALL SQUAT
(AGAINST WALL)

Reps: 20

Description/Notes:

1 Stand upright facing away from a wall, position the ball between your back and the wall, so you are leaning against it.

2 Perform a normal deep squat rolling the ball up and down the wall. Use weight to increase difficulty level.

For a video of this exercise, visit:

www.youtube.com/watch?v=ydVHCRhEnj8

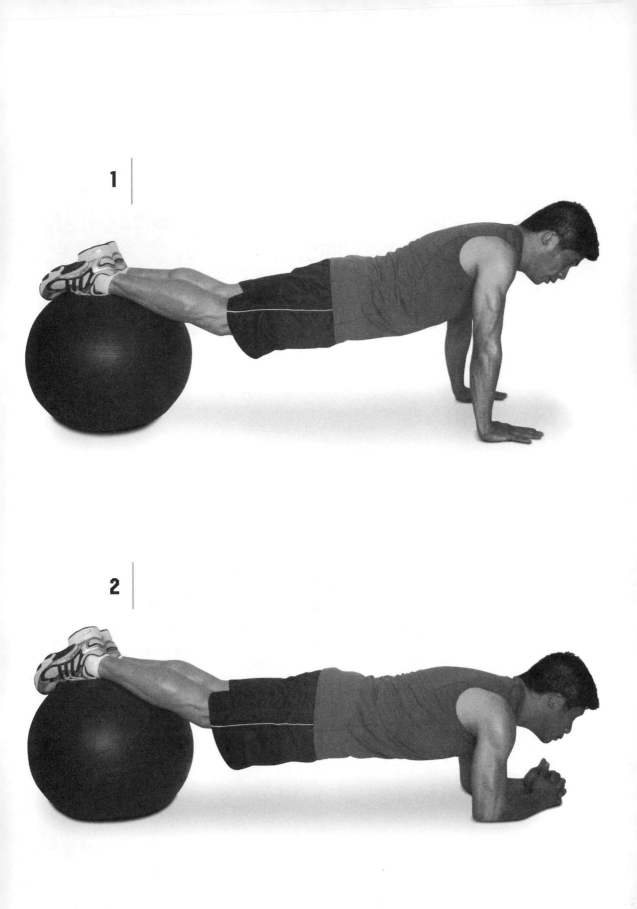

SWISS BALL "PLANK"
(FEET ON SWISS BALL)

Reps: 1 minute

Description/Notes:

1 Assume the push-up position with your feet balanced on top of the ball.

2 Then adopt the "plank" position by dropping your elbows and forearms onto the floor. Hold this position for 1 minute.

For a video of this exercise, visit:

www.youtube.com/watch?v=SXh6psb0FbO

(In the video, the man adds a Bosu ball for extra difficulty.)

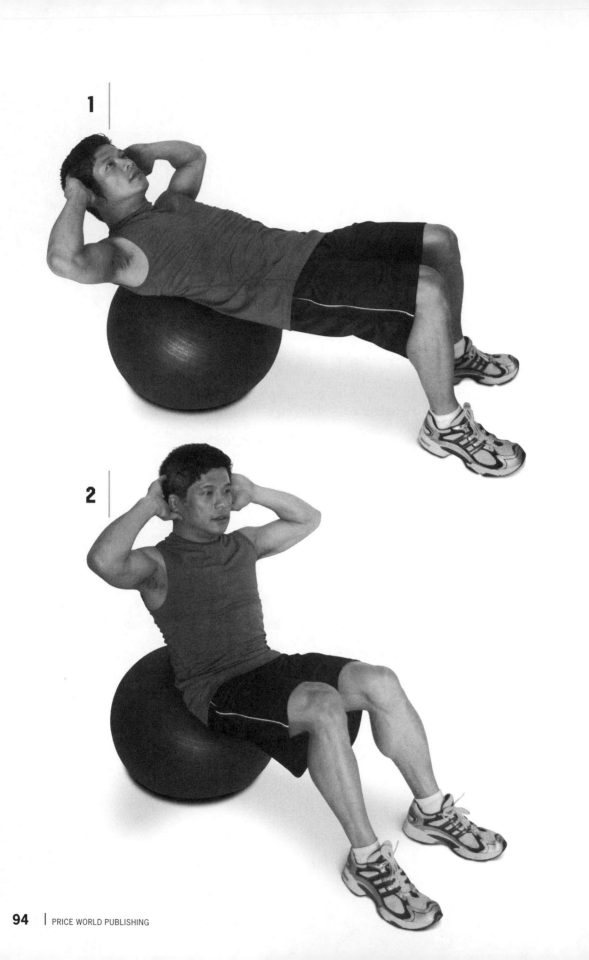

SWISS BALL CRUNCH
(LIE ON BALL)

Reps: 20

Description/Notes:

1 | Lie with your back on the Swiss ball, feet flat on the floor, knees bent to 90 degrees.

2 | Engage you abdominals and crunch up so your upper back is no longer in contact with the ball. Return slowly to the starting position.

For a video of this exercise, visit:

www.youtube.com/watch?v=05MebP8rYWQ

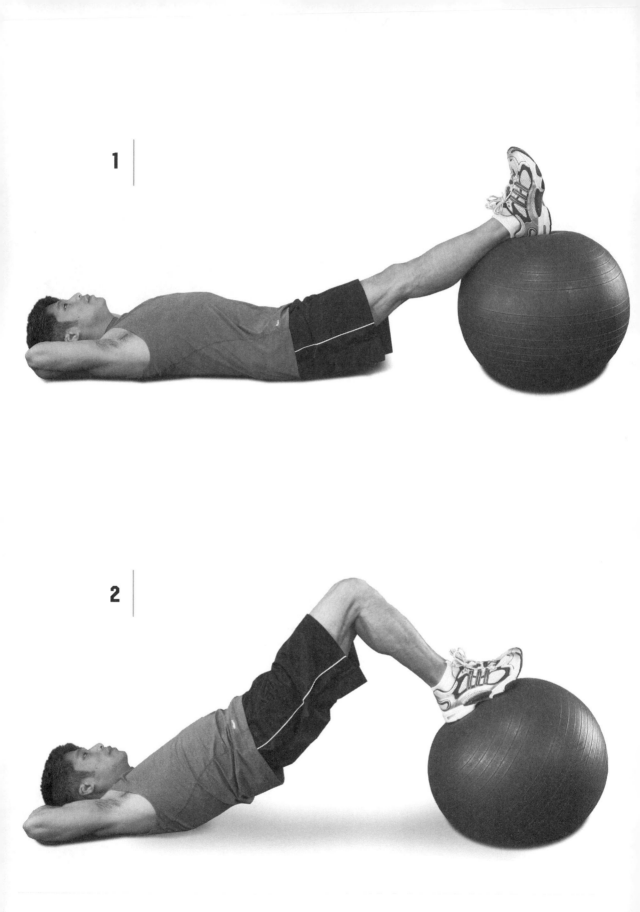

SWISS BALL
HAMSTRING CURL

Reps: 20

Description/Notes:

1 | Lie face up on the floor, feet balanced on the Swiss ball with your body completely straight.

2 | Roll the ball toward you using your feet until your knees are bent to 90 degrees, at this point only your upper back and head should be in contact with the floor.

Increase difficultly by working each leg individually, i.e., only having one leg in contact with the ball.

For a video of this exercise, visit:

www.youtube.com/watch?v=czf-1snzG2c

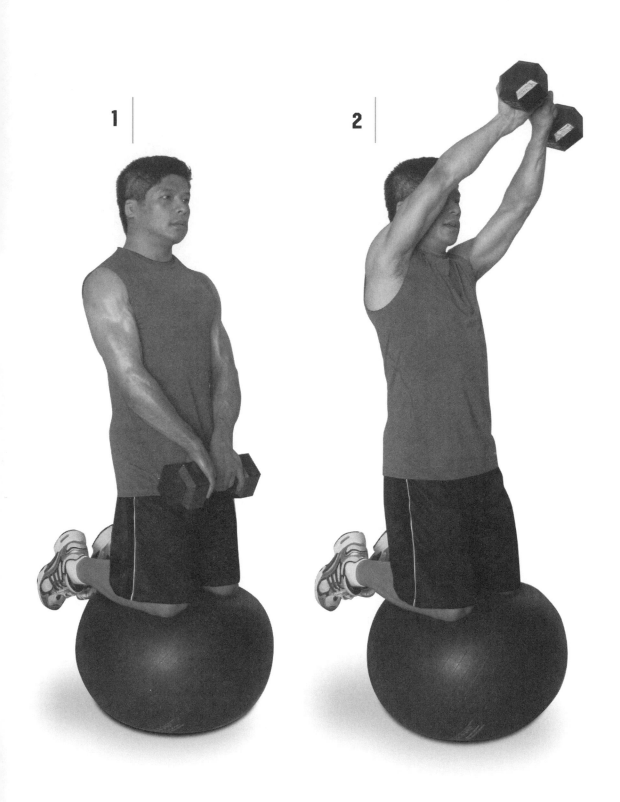

REVERSE WOODCHOPS
KNEELING ON SWISS BALL

Reps: 10 on each side

Description/Notes:

1 Start by kneeling on the Swiss ball and getting into a position where you can maintain your balance.

2 Once stable, take the dumbbell in both hands and perform a chopping motion from high right to low left. Repeat on the other side (high left to low right).

For a video of this exercise, visit:

www.youtube.com/watch?v=XgqRQP7lfbs

(In the video, the man uses a machine, which is just as effective.)

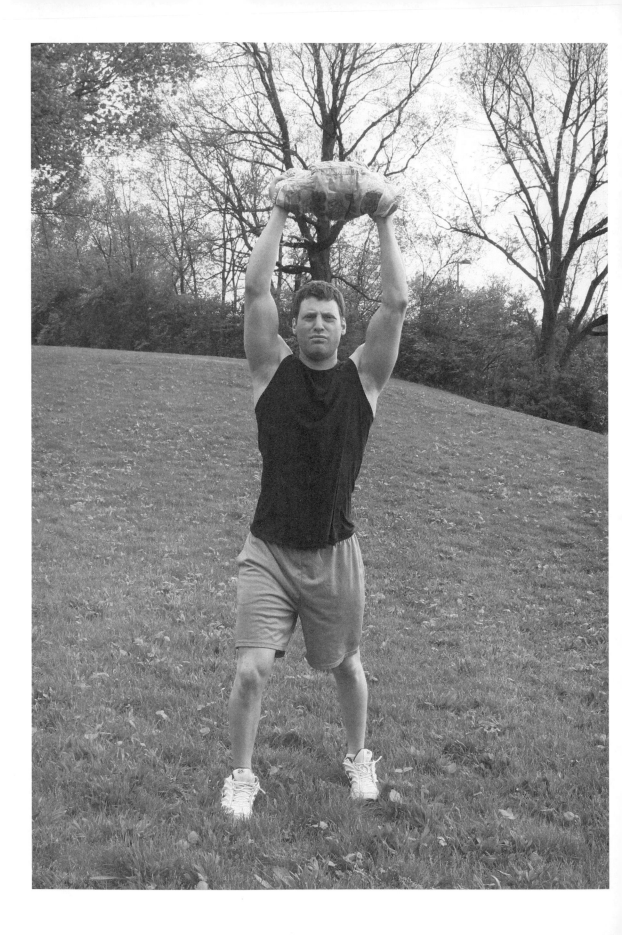

Hill Workout

A good hill workout is a great alternative to the gym or a boring run. However, these workouts are not for the fainthearted, they are a true test of both aerobic and anaerobic fitness. Anyone wanting to increase their explosive power, particularly in their legs, should consider putting a hill circuit in their training routine.

If you don't live near a hill, there is still no excuse for avoiding this circuit because a long set of stairs will do just as well. Ideally, you should look for a hill with a relatively sharp incline–somewhere around 10 percent will do fine. Of course, if you feel up to it, find a steeper incline and increase the difficulty level. To perform the circuit correctly, you need 40 meters/yards of hill. Before you start, mark out this distance to avoid cheating later on.

Just to give your circuit that additional "spice," we have added a sandbag. We definitely recommend you get a sandbag as they are cheap, versatile, and easy to find. You can pick up a sandbag and some sand at any builder's supply or do-it-yourself store for next to nothing. If money is no object, consider investing in a Powerbag.

SANDBAG CLEAN AND PRESS

HILL SPRINT WITH SANDBAG

SQUAT WITH SANDBAG

HILL SPRINT WITH OVERHEAD SANDBAG THROWS

BURPEES WITH A JUMPING JACK

UPHILL DUCK WALKS WITH SANDBAG

PUSH-UPS (FACING DOWNHILL)

Equipment Required

One sandbag or equivalent weighing between 10-20kgs (25-45 pounds).

Instructions

Carry out 3 sets of the 7 exercises.

Take a 2-minute rest between sets.

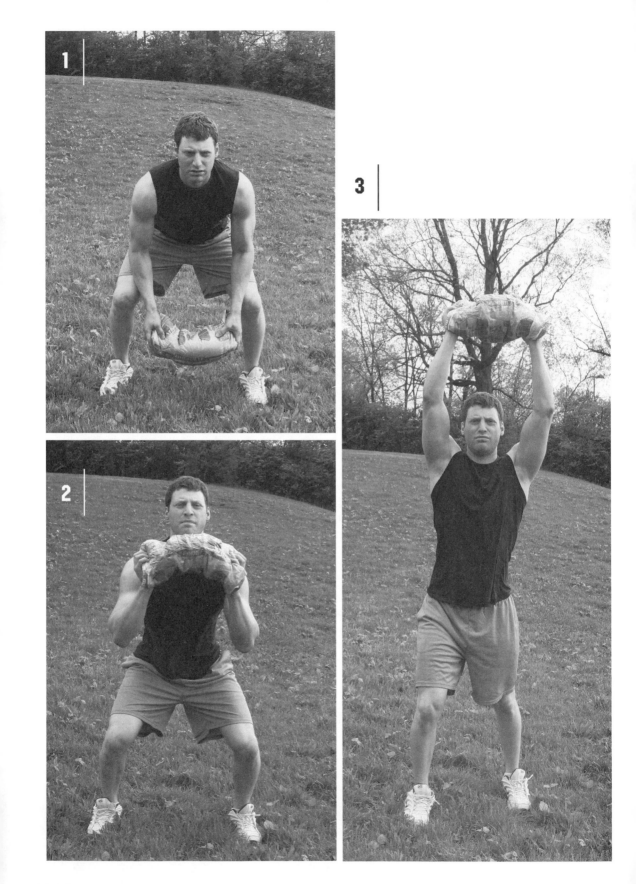

SANDBAG CLEAN AND PRESS

Reps: 20

Description/Notes:

1	Stand in front of the sandbag, back straight, knees bent.
2	Grab it with both hands and clean it in one dynamic motion, and then press it above your head.

To perform a sandbag clean, pull the sandbag up explosively, and when it reaches your mid thighs, shrug it up while simultaneously dropping yourself beneath it and performing what is effectively a reverse curl. Return the bag to the ground under control to complete 1 repetition.

1 **2**

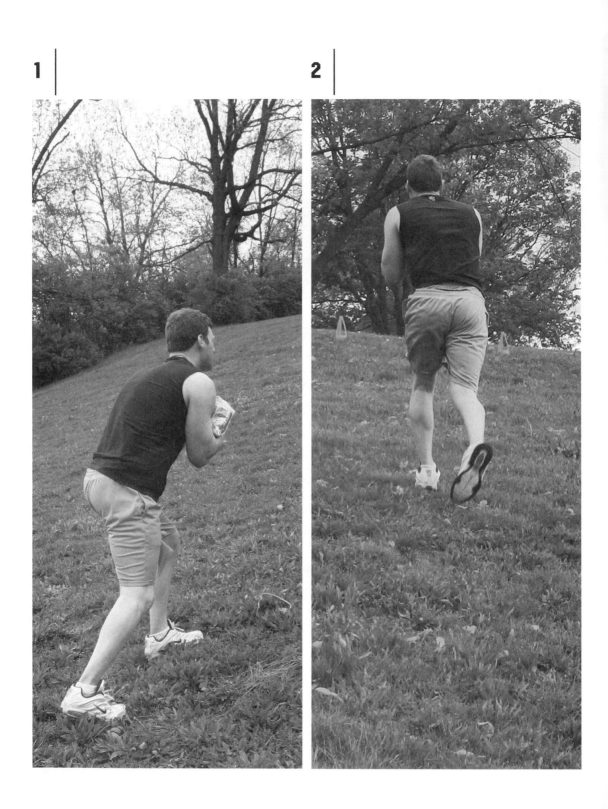

HILL SPRINT WITH SANDBAG

Reps: 2

Description/Notes:

1 | Stand at the bottom of the hill in front of the 40-meter/yard marker you marked out earlier. Hold the sandbag in both hands close to your chest.

2 | Sprint up the hill to your marker and slowly jog back down. Repeat this twice for each set.

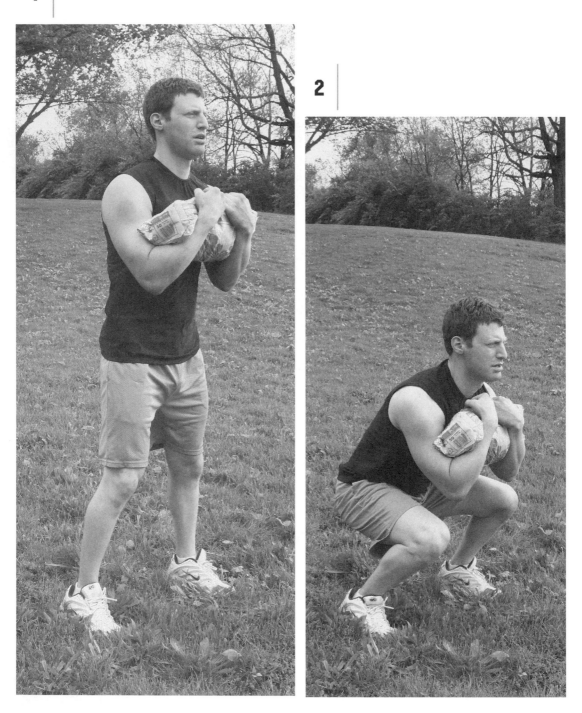

SQUAT WITH SANDBAG

Reps: 20

Description/Notes:

1	Hold the sandbag in both hands close to your chest.
2	Perform a deep squat (knees bent to 90 degrees) making sure to keep your back straight. Return to upright starting position under control.

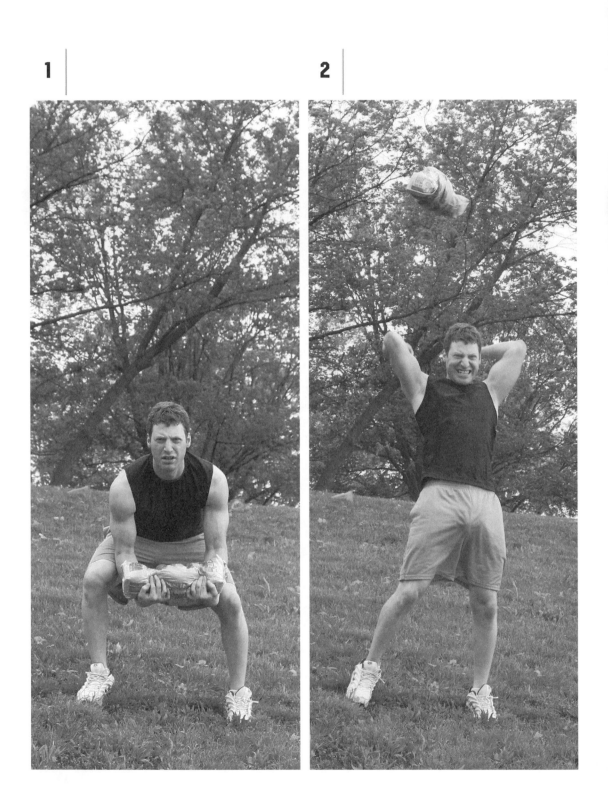

HILL SPRINT WITH OVERHEAD SANDBAG THROWS

Reps: 2

Description/Notes:

1 Stand at the bottom of the hill in front of the 40-meter/yard marker. Face down hill.

2 Hold the sandbag in front of you and throw it backwards, over your head as far as you can (i.e. uphill). Then sprint uphill to where the bag landed, pick it up, and throw it over your head again. Repeat this until you reach your other 40-meter marker. Slowly jog back down with the bag. Repeat this twice for each set.

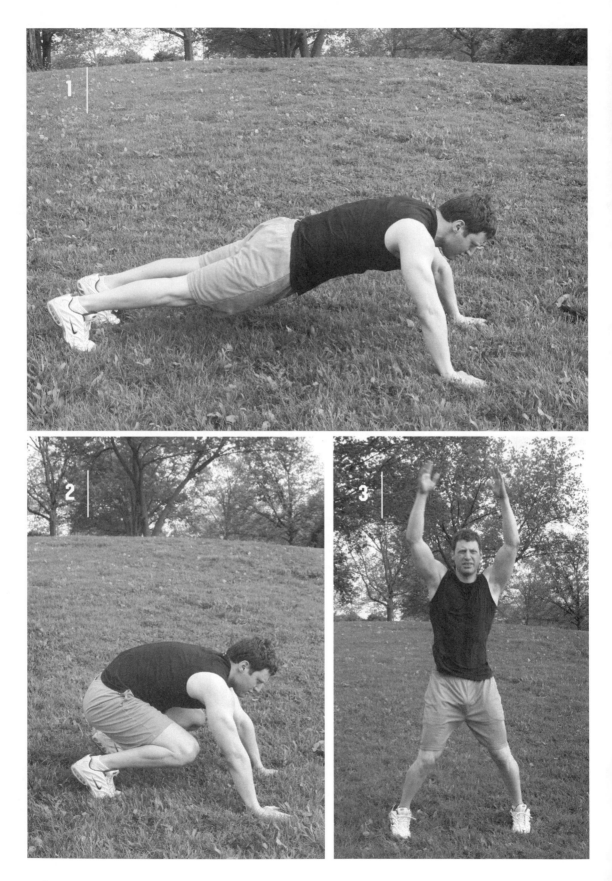

BURPEES WITH A JUMPING JACK

Reps: 20

Description/Notes:

1 | To perform a burpee, start in the push-up position.

2 | Bring your knees to chest.

3 | Then perform a jumping jack and return to your original position.

(Bag not required for this exercise).

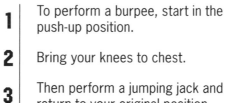

For a video of this exercise, visit:

www.youtube.com/watch?v=c_Dq_NCzj8M

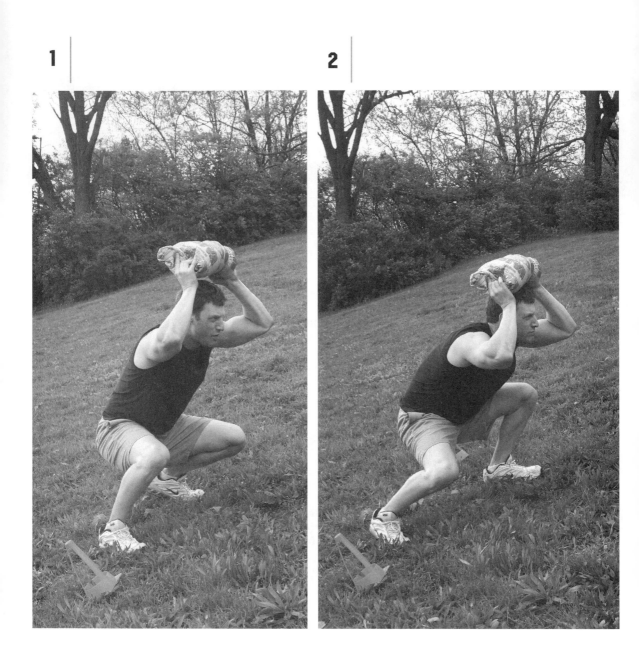

UPHILL DUCK WALKS WITH SANDBAG

Reps: 1

Description/Notes:

1 | Stand at the bottom of the hill in front of the 40-meter/yard marker. Assume the squat position holding the sandbag above your head.

2 | Maintaining the squat position "walk" up the hill to your other marker. Slowly jog back down.

See the video for more pointers on technique.

For a video of this exercise, visit:

www.youtube.com/watch?v=CtdxTeOEpFM

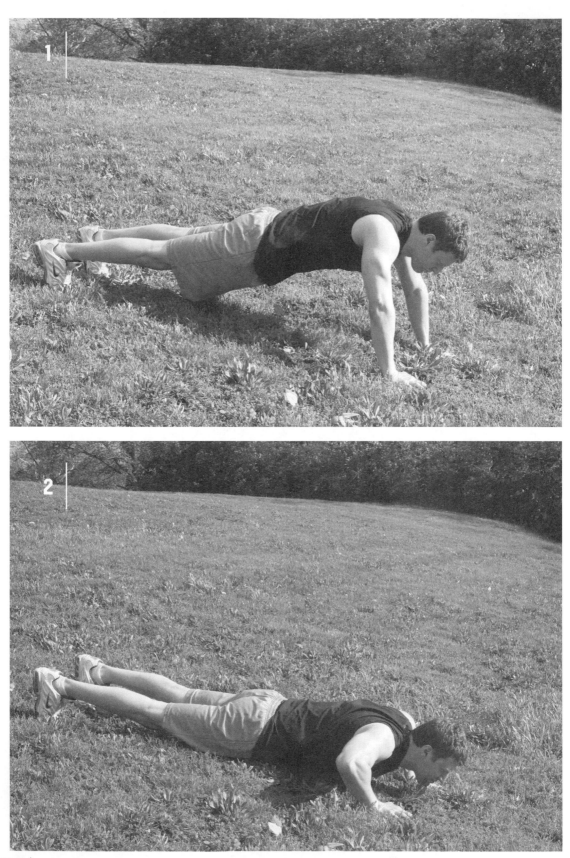

PUSH-UPS
(FACING DOWNHILL)

Reps: 20

Description/Notes:

1 | Face downhill and adopt the push-up position. You should be facing downhill with your legs on higher ground than your arms.

2 | Carry out 20 normal push-ups.

(Bag not required for this exercise, unless you want to put it on your back for extra weight.)

Multi-Machine

This multi-machine gym circuit is a quick "all-action" high-intensity session, perfect for someone in a hurry or someone who needs to fit a workout into a lunch break. All exercises should be completed with 100 percent effort.

Try timing the whole circuit and keeping a record of times in a logbook. Always aim to improve on your best time. www.gyminee.com

If your gym doesn't have all the necessary equipment or is too busy, you could try changing the order of the circuit to suit you more or, as a last resort, substitute some of the exercises for others in this book.

CYCLE

ROW

LAT PULL-DOWN

SIT-UPS

PUSH-UPS

STEP-UPS

SIT-UPS

SHOULDER PRESS

UPHILL RUN

BENCH PRESS

Equipment Required

Various equipment, most of which should be found in normal gym: exercise bike; rowing machine; treadmill; Lat Pull-down Machine; two dumbbells (weight load depends upon your ability and size); bench (24 inches above the floor); barbell; and two plates (weight load depends upon your ability and size).

Instructions

Carry out 1 set of the 10 exercises. Maximum speed.

No rest between sets, make sure to time the set.

CYCLE

1.6km

Use an exercise bike so
you can keep an eye on the
distance (1.6km = 1 mile).

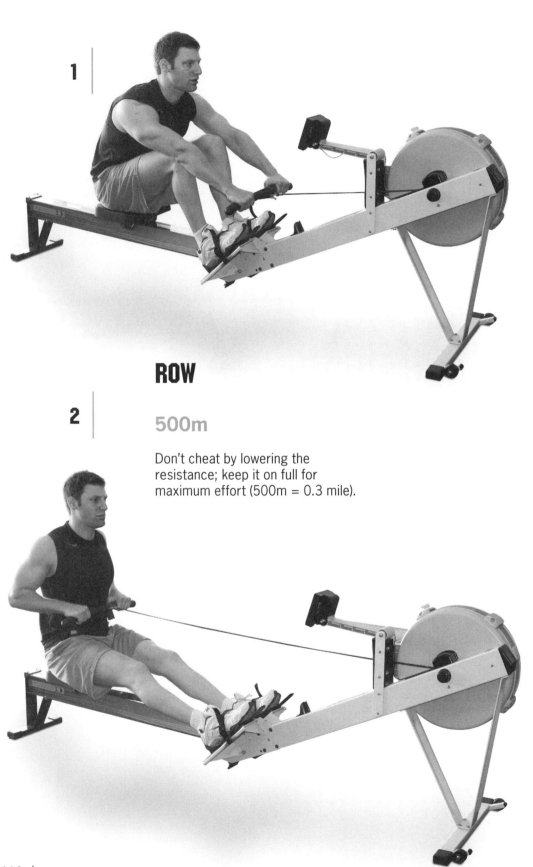

1

ROW

2

500m

Don't cheat by lowering the resistance; keep it on full for maximum effort (500m = 0.3 mile).

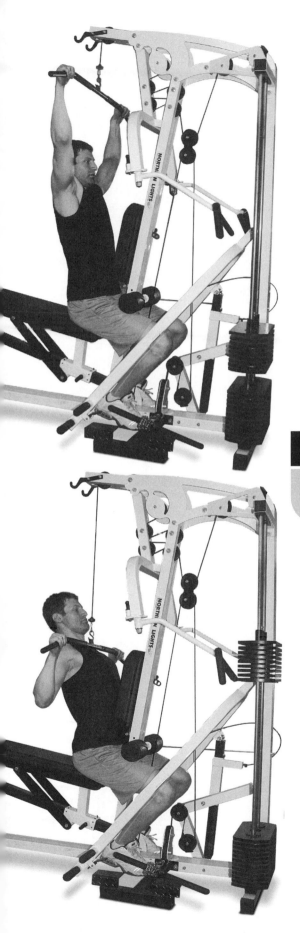

LAT PULL-DOWN

Reps: 40

Use a machine. Start with a relatively light weight. The aim is to do 40 reps in one go. If the weight you select is too easy, increase it. Don't worry if you can't do it straightaway; break it up into smaller sets.

For a video of this exercise, visit:

www.youtube.com/watch?v=d_N6Tq5F9vA

1

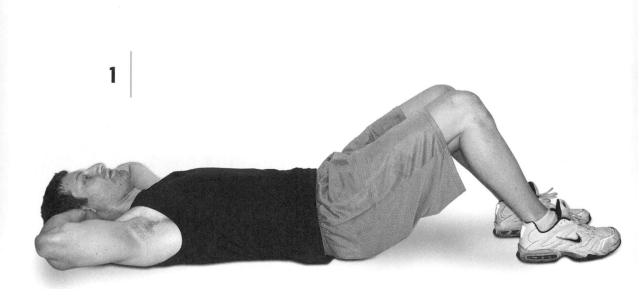

SIT-UPS

Reps: 60

Hands on side of head,
chest all the way up to
knees. Again, aim to finish
in one go without a break.

2

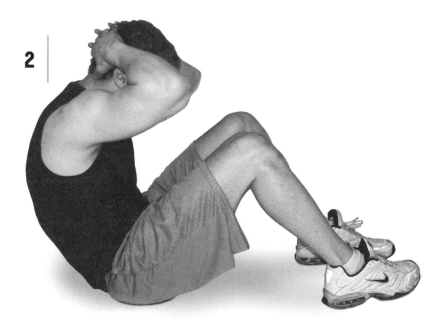

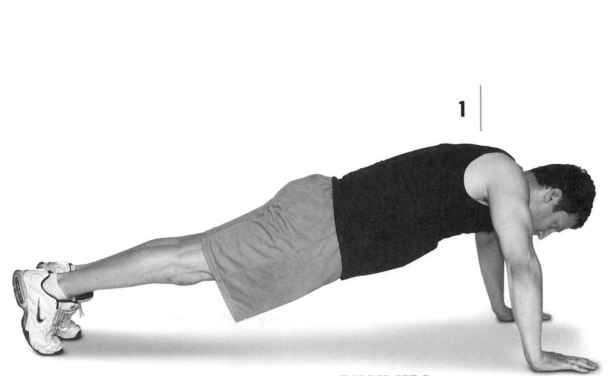

1

PUSH-UPS

Reps: 50

Adopt the push-up position on
the floor. Keep legs together.
Bend arm to 90 degree angle.
Aim to finish in one go without
a break.

2

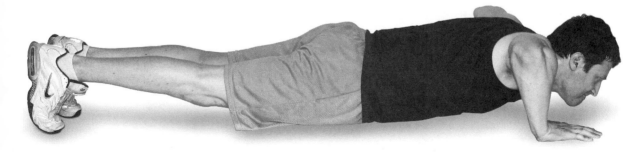

STEP-UPS

Reps: 100

Holding a dumbbell in each arm, perform 100 step-ups onto a bench approximately 24 inches off the floor. Do 50 reps on one leg then change legs.

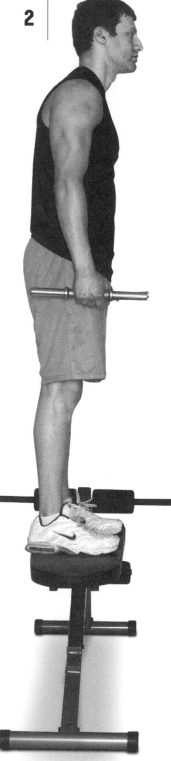

2

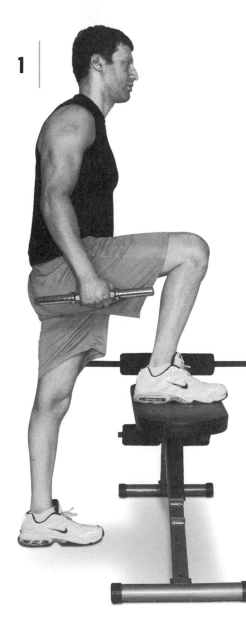

1

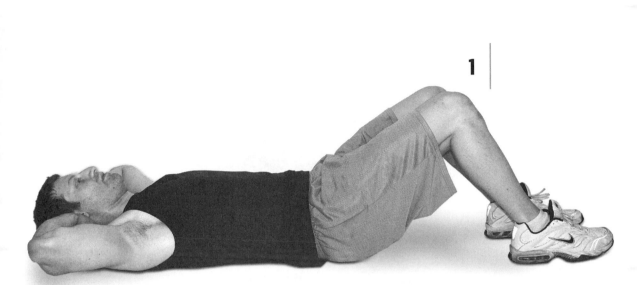

1

SIT-UPS

Reps: 60

Hands on side of head,
chest all the way up to
knees. Again, aim to finish
in one go without a break.

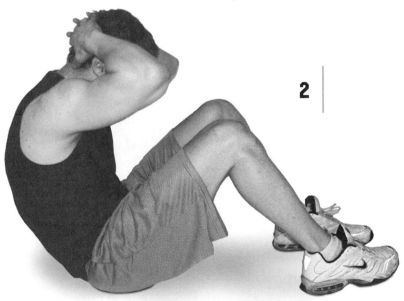

2

1

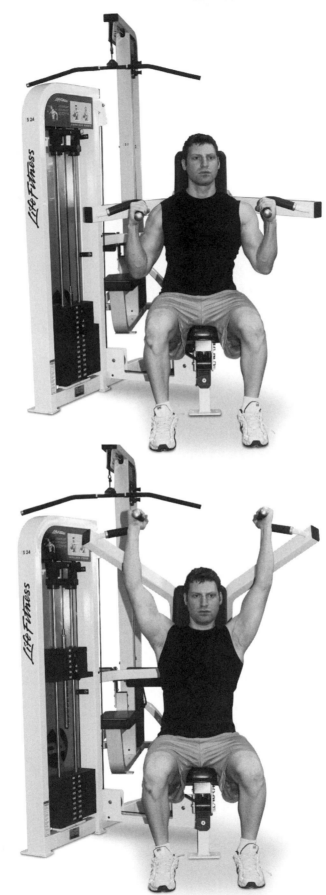

2

SHOULDER PRESS

Reps: 40

Use a machine. Start with a
relatively light weight. If it's too
easy, increase the weight.

For a video of this exercise, visit:

www.youtube.com/watch?v=cr2j5Wigopw

UPHILL RUN

800M

Use a treadmill
and incline it to
10 percent.
Maximum effort
to finish as quickly
as possible.

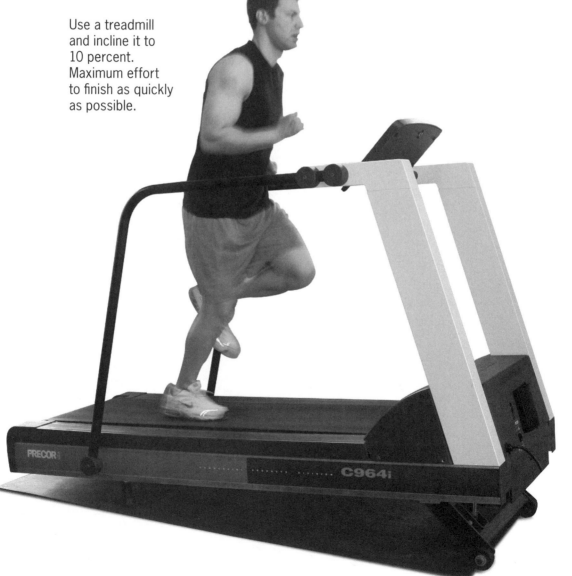

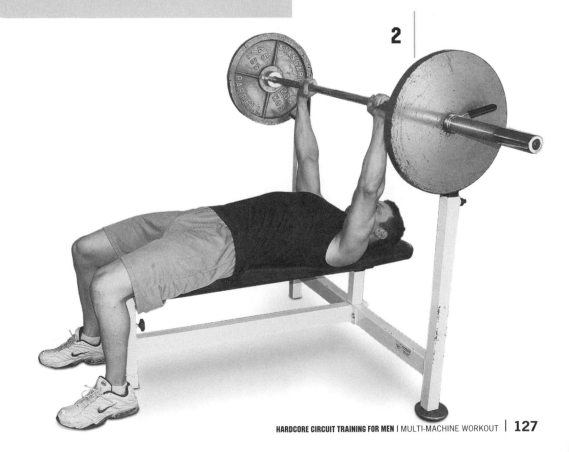

1

BENCH PRESS

Reps: 40

Ideally use a barbell for the bench press. Start relatively light. If you start out too light, increase the weight.

For a video of this exercise, visit:

www.youtube.com/watch?v=wOnP_oAXUMA

2

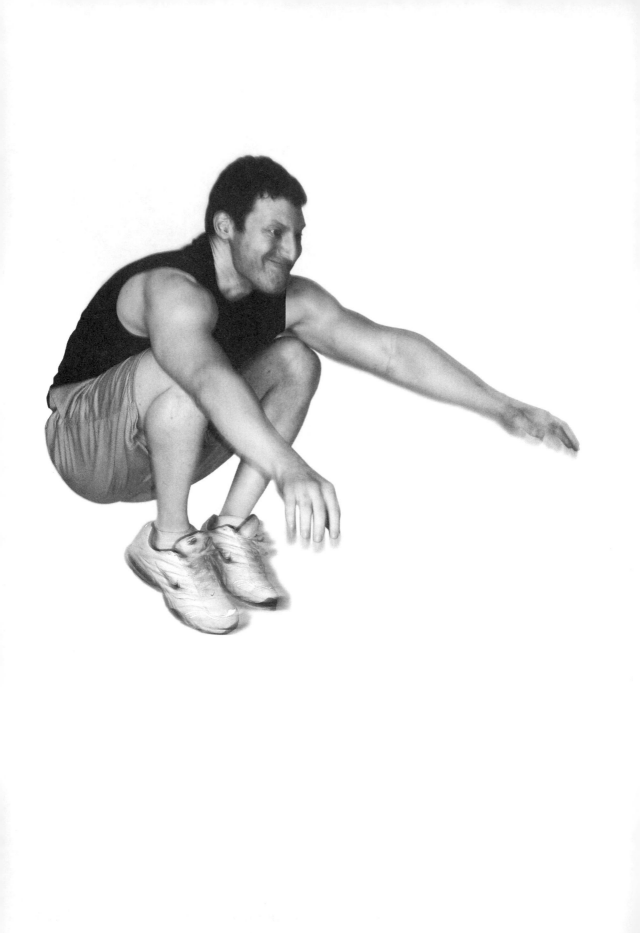

The 4 Miler

The 4 Miler (6.4km) is an extremely uncomplicated but effective circuit. It is ideal if you wish to improve your aerobic fitness. It is a short fast run broken up by a few small exercise circuits. As with the multi-machine workout, it is ideal for someone in a hurry or to fit into a lunch break.

The run is a "run" and not a jog. Make sure you are working between 70 percent and 80 percent of your working heart rate (see the introduction to calculate your working heart rate).

If you wish, you can increase the difficulty by extending the distance of the run to five or six miles.

BURPEES WITH A "SPIDERMAN" PUSH-UP

TUCK JUMPS

DYNAMIC "CLAP" PUSH-UPS

SIT-UPS

Equipment Required

None

Instructions

Four-mile run. Run approximately 1 mile then complete 1 set of the following 4 exercises. Without a rest, run the next mile and again complete another 1 set of the 4 exercises. Repeat until the end of the run.

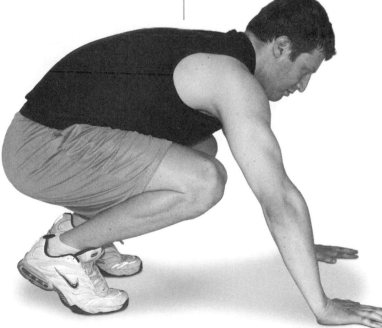

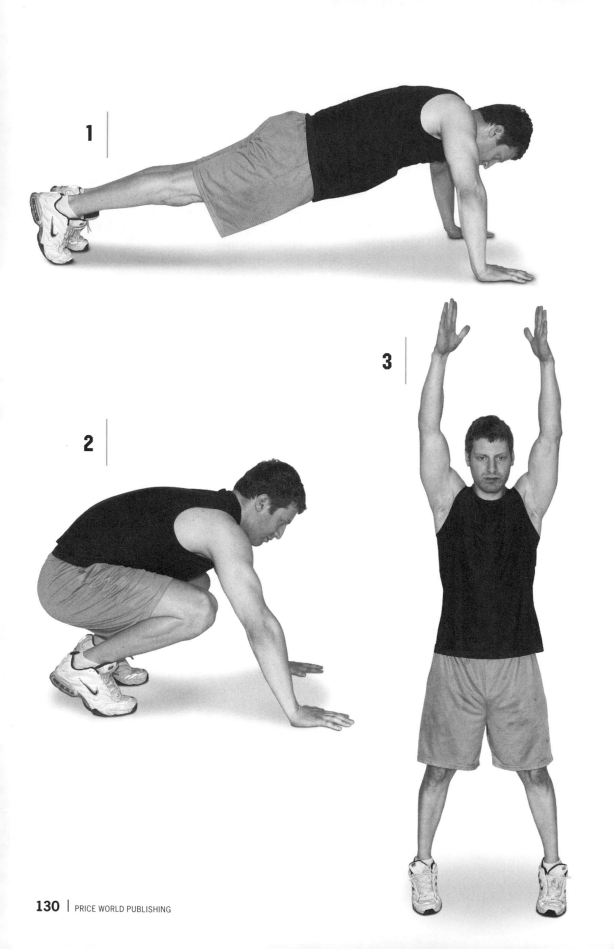

BURPEES WITH A "SPIDERMAN" PUSH-UP

Reps: 20

Description/Notes:

1 | Start in the push-up position. Perform a "spiderman" push-up.

2 | Then bring your knees into your chest.

3 | Stand up, and perform a dynamic jump. Return to your original position to complete the exercise.

For a video of this exercise, visit:

www.youtube.com/watch?v=eHbJoeA1I4E

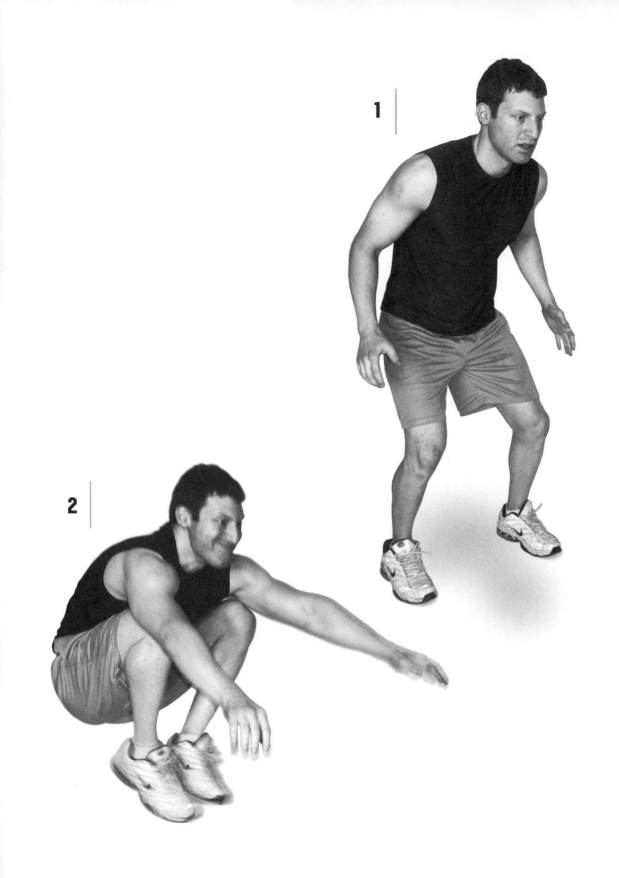

TUCK JUMPS

Reps: 25

Description/Notes:

1 | A basic but effective exercise. Stand upright.

2 | Jump off the floor, and bring your knees into your chest. Straighten your legs out again before landing the jump.

For a video of this exercise, visit:

www.youtube.com/watch?v=Q2yH1vixV4g

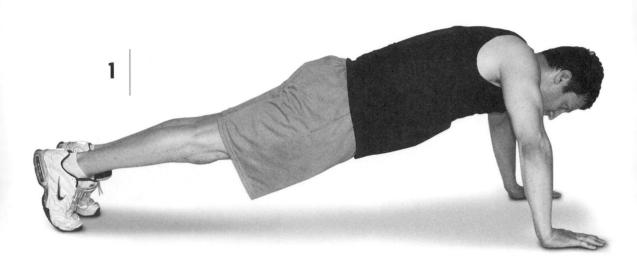

1

DYNAMIC "CLAP" PUSH-UPS

Reps: 15

Description/Notes:

1 | Start in the push-up position.

2 | Hands leave the floor as you push off. Quickly bring them together (hence "clap") before returning hands to the floor.

2

For a video of this exercise, visit:

www.youtube.com/watch?v=ti0ugruVaGl

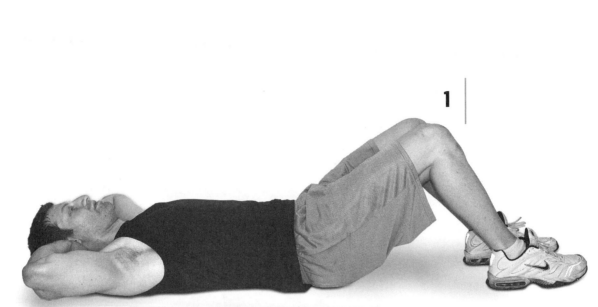

1

SIT-UPS

Reps: 30

Description/Notes:

1 Keep hands on side of head.

2 Chest should come all the way up to knees.

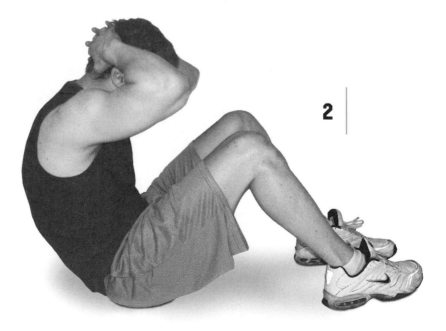

2

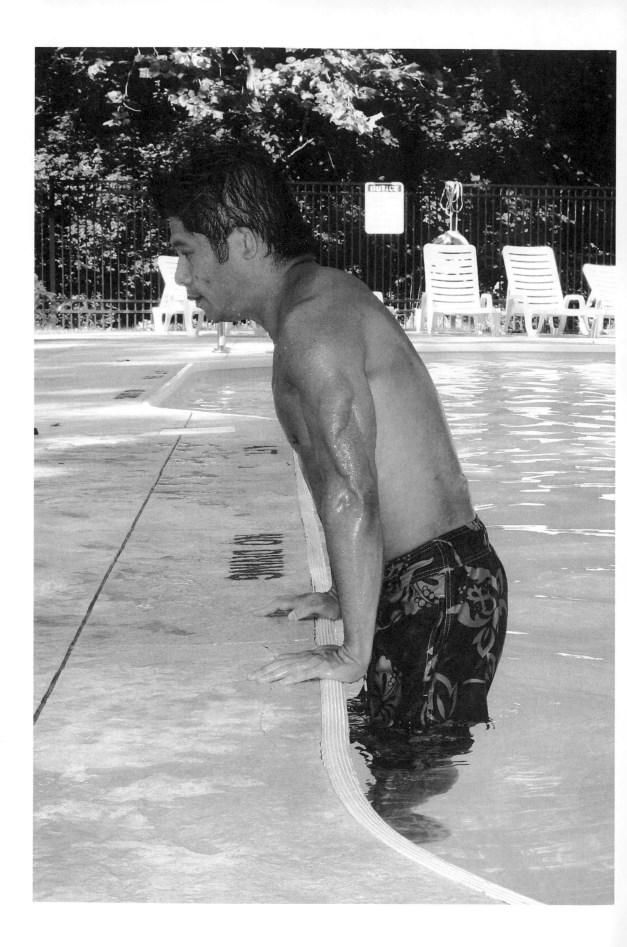

Swim Circuit

Swimming is great exercise. It's low impact, thereby reducing stress on your joints, and at the same time, water still provides plenty of resistance to tone your muscles and improve fitness. If you have access to a pool, seriously consider making swimming a regular feature in your training routine.

The most common complaint we hear about swimming is that it's boring. Monotonous lengths of the pool using the same stroke can get tedious. We believe the key to making it more interesting is to break down your swim into sets. You could try using different strokes or different drills. The technique we have used for this circuit is to add in some exercises with the swimming. It certainly eliminates the boredom factor.

We appreciate that not everyone is a competent swimmer or has access to a nearby pool. However, it is worth making the effort to fit swimming in somewhere in your routine. If you have trouble swimming, just reduce the number of lengths in the circuit, changing it to suit your ability. If you want to improve you swimming, try the total immersion teaching method–**www.totalimmersion.net/**– it is very effective.

BREAST STROKE

FRONT DIPS

FREESTYLE
(FRONT CRAWL)

PUSH-UPS

BUTTERFLY STROKE

SIT-UPS

FREESTYLE
(FRONT CRAWL)

Equipment Required

None, except maybe some Speedos and goggles.

Instructions

Carry out 4 sets of the 7 exercises.

Take a 30-second rest between sets.

BREASTSTROKE

250m

Work at 75% effort for 250m (10 lengths of a 25m pool).

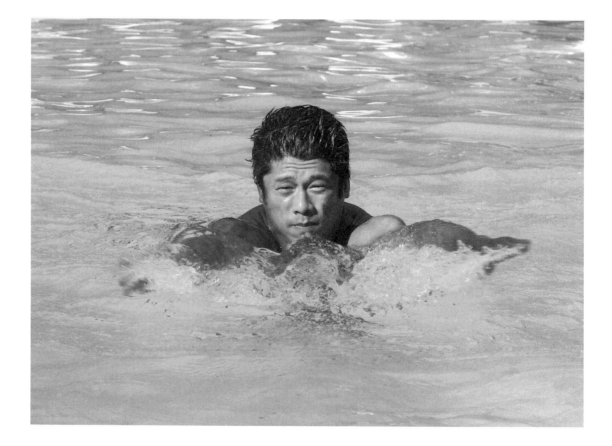

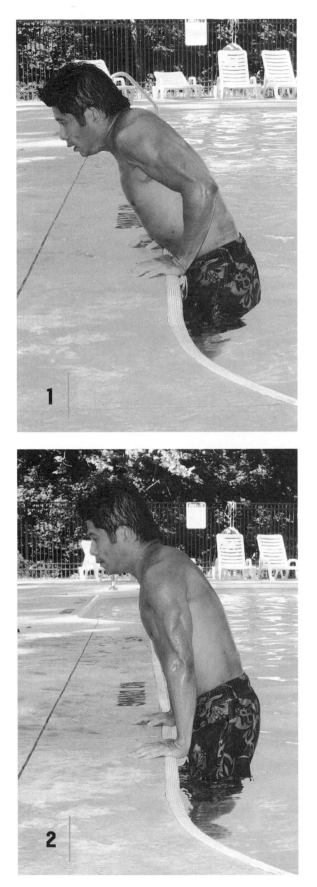

FRONT DIPS

Reps: 30

Description/Notes:

1 | Face the side of the pool putting both hands on the edge, feet should not be touching the bottom of the pool.

2 | Push up, lifting your torso out of the water until your arms are straight then return under control.

FREESTYLE (FRONT CRAWL)
200M

100% effort. Sprint for 200m (8 lengths of a 25m pool).

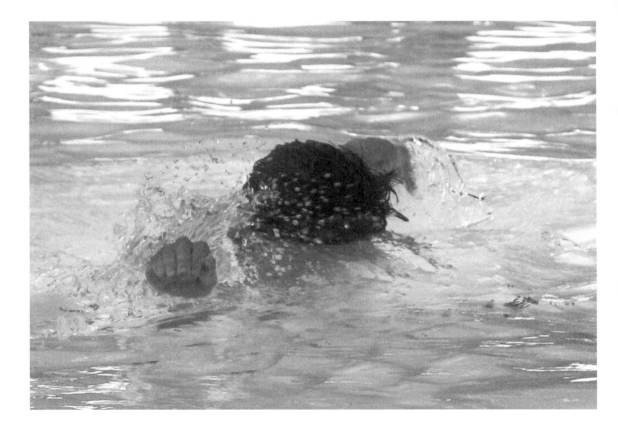

PUSH-UPS

Reps: 25

Get out of the pool and carry out 25 standard push-ups by the side. Take care not to slip on the wet surface.

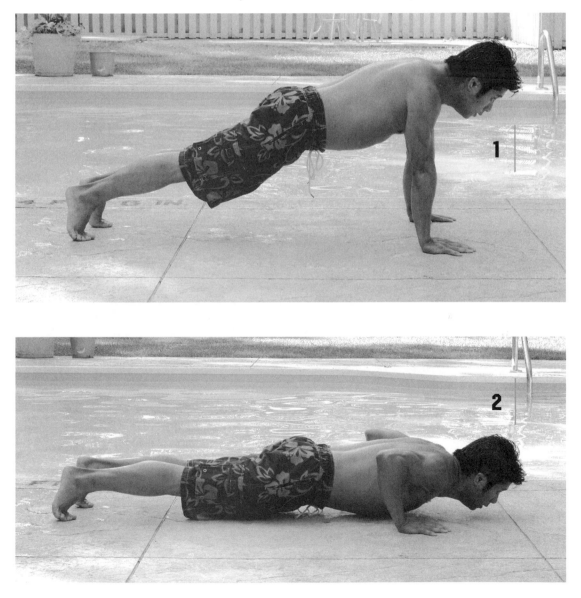

BUTTERFLY STROKE

50M

100% effort. Sprint for 50m (2 lengths of a 25m pool).

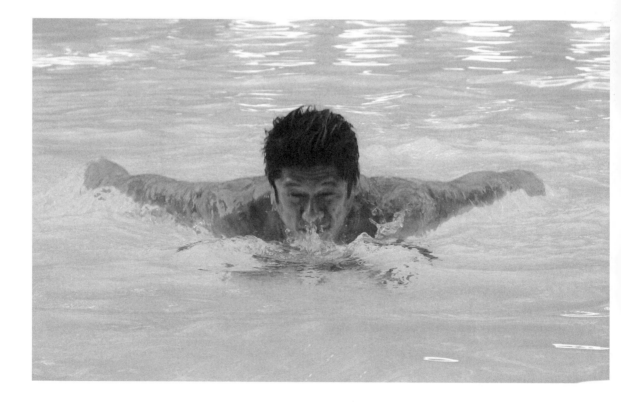

SIT-UPS

50

Hands on side of head, chest all the way up to knees.

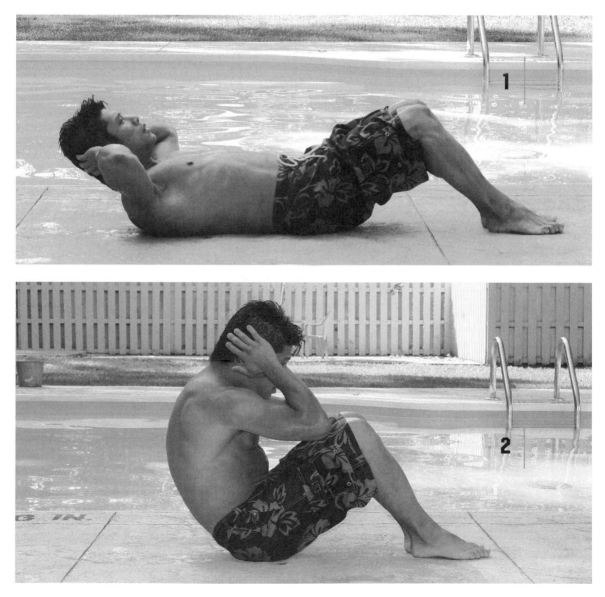

FREESTYLE (FRONT CRAWL)
200M

Again 100% effort to finish the circuit.
Sprint for 200m (8 lengths of a 25m pool).

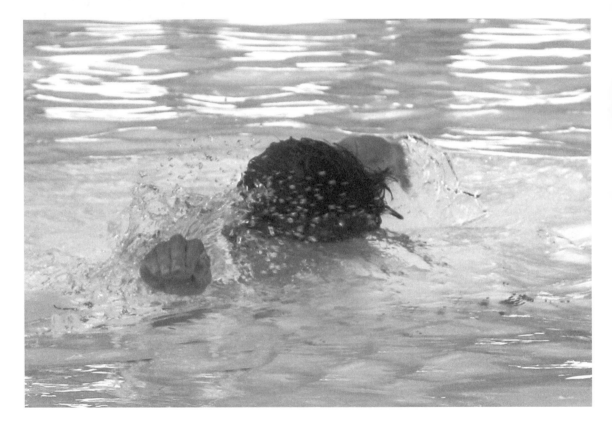

PART III | Fitness & Strength Tests

Testing your fitness and strength on a regular basis is extremely important (and not just because you might get bragging rights over your friends). By regularly testing, you can establish whether your training is working and that you are making steps toward achieving your goals. Use the following three tests to measure your strength and fitness.

The Multistage Fitness Test

The multistage fitness test, more commonly known as the "Beep Test," is perhaps the best known and most used fitness test of all. It is still considered THE benchmark of aerobic fitness. You can find out more about it at **www.en.wikipedia.org/wiki/Multi-stage_fitness_test.**

Feared and respected in equal measure, it is a maximal test that gets progressively harder. Originally, it was designed to help estimate your VO2 Max, or in plain English, the maximum amount of oxygen your body can uptake and use during exercise.

In essence, the test involves running between two markers set 20 meters/yards apart. Your runs between these two markers must be synchronized with a prerecorded audio track of "beeps." You will need access to a CD player or equivalent to carry out the test. The audio recording can be downloaded for free at **www.runtheplanet.com/img/trainingracing/ training/bleep_test.mp3**.

As the test progresses, the time between the "beeps" reduces so you have less time to reach the marker, and therefore, it becomes harder and harder. The test finishes when you either reach the end of the recording (not easy) or can no longer reach the marker before a "beep" sounds.

Remember your score (i.e., the level you reach) and use it as a benchmark to measure yourself against next time you take the test.

The "300"

The "300" or "Spartan Workout" was developed by Mark Twight, the founder of Gym Jones (www.gymjones.com). It was used to test the cast of the Frank Miller film *300*, during their grueling training program. Mark was kind enough to let us reprint his workout here.

The "300" is extremely high intensity and requires strength, power, endurance, and aerobic fitness. Take a look at this video for a full demonstration:
www.youtube.com/watch?v=ggiYjRelWgc.

The "300" is measured by the time it takes you to complete all seven exercises. Obviously, the less time you take, the better your score. Although you should note that time is only a meaningful measurement if loads are the same and, more importantly, if range of motion is the same for every person and every repetition. With this in mind, your time for the circuit is not a score in the sense of being able to compare yourself to another individual. Each of our bodies is different—a tall guy has to move the bar on a dead lift exercise further than a short guy.

Use your score (time) as a way to benchmark your own performance and improve your fitness.

This is how Mark described
The "300" to us in his own words:

When describing the workout, it is more accurate to say that it requires strength, power endurance and aerobic fitness, as it is generally a person's inability to continuously produce the power needed to do the movement over and over and over.

Although time is the measurement we used, the stopwatch is only meaningful if loads are the same (I've seen many scaled versions using lighter weights and even elastic resistance bands), and more importantly range of motion is the same for every person and every rep. If the chest doesn't hit the floor on the push-up, the rep does not count. If the whole head does not rise above the bar on the pull-up the rep does not count - no matter how fast it is done.

And finally, one's time for the circuit is not a score in the sense of comparing oneself to another individual. If all reps are done to standard and the prescribed loads are used (these parameters are fixed) then the time, the only variable, tells us something. The less time one takes, the higher the power output, the greater the fitness; a fast time means the athlete is more than equal to the task. Using time to compare between individuals could only be accurate or meaningful if their bodies are the same: the guy who is 6'3" tall has to move the bar further during the deadlift than the guy who is 5'7" tall ... no comparison.

Equipment Required

Pull-up bar or equivalent; one barbell; two plates (weight load depends upon your ability and size); one kettlebell or dumbbell (weight loads depend upon your ability and size).

Instructions

Seven exercises, total of 300 repetitions in the minimum amount of time possible. The "300" is timed, so ideally you shouldn't take a rest between exercises.

OVERHAND PULL-UPS

DEAD LIFTS

PUSH-UPS

BOX JUMPS

FLOOR WIPERS

SINGLE-HAND KETTLEBELL CLEAN AND PRESS

OVERHAND PULL-UPS

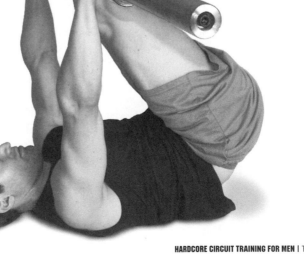

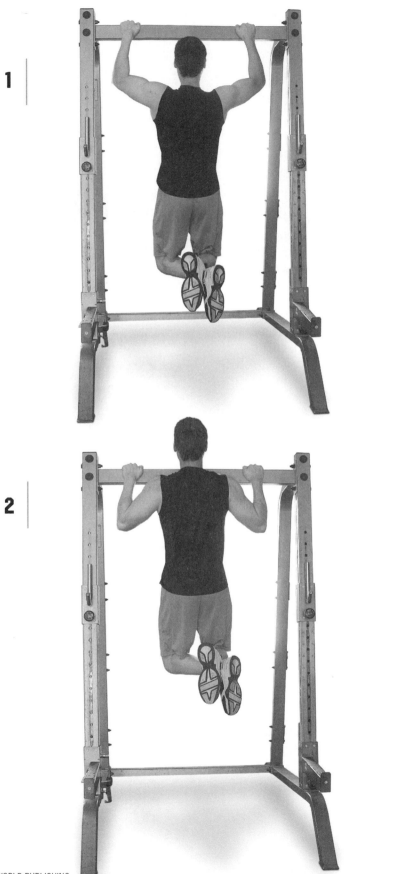

OVERHAND PULL-UPS

Reps: 25

Description/Notes:

1 | Find a pull-up bar high enough so your feet don't touch the floor. Assume an overhand grip on the bar.

2 | Pull up your body so your chin is above the bar then return under control until your arms are full extended.

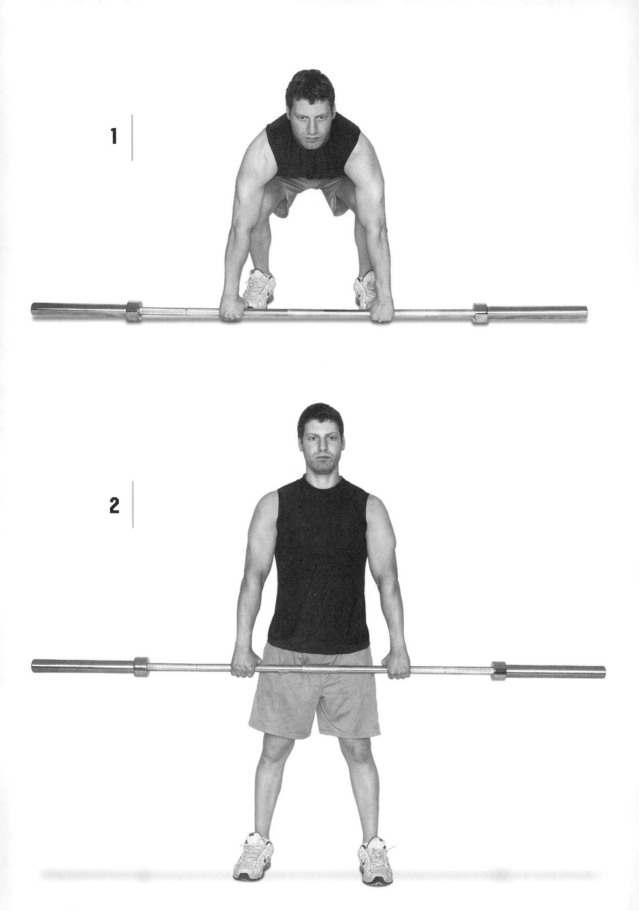

DEAD LIFTS

Reps: 50

Description/Notes:

1 | You need a barbell with two plates, 1 on either side. Keeping your back straight, bend your knees and grip the bar with both hands.

2 | Lift the bar from the floor and straighten your knees until you are standing fully upright, then return the bar to the floor under control.

Technique is important with this exercise to avoid injury. Make sure to take a look at the video for tips.

1

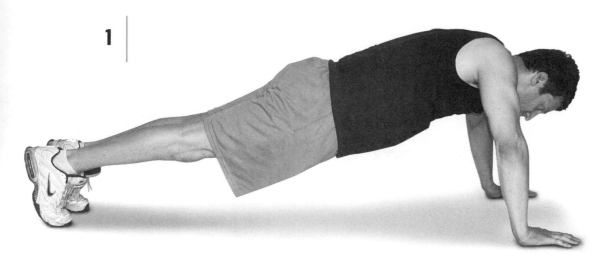

PUSH-UPS

Reps: 50

Description/Notes:

1 | Adopt the push-up position on the floor. Keep legs together.

2 | Bend arms to 90-degree angle. Aim to finish in one go without a break.

2

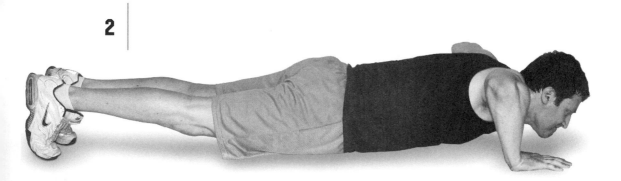

BOX JUMPS

Reps: 50

Description/Notes:

1 Find a bench at least 24 inches off the floor. Stand up, facing toward the bench.

2 Jump (using both legs, keeping them together) onto the bench and then back onto the floor. Do not step onto the bench.

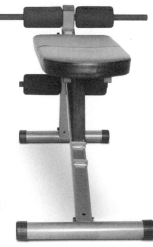

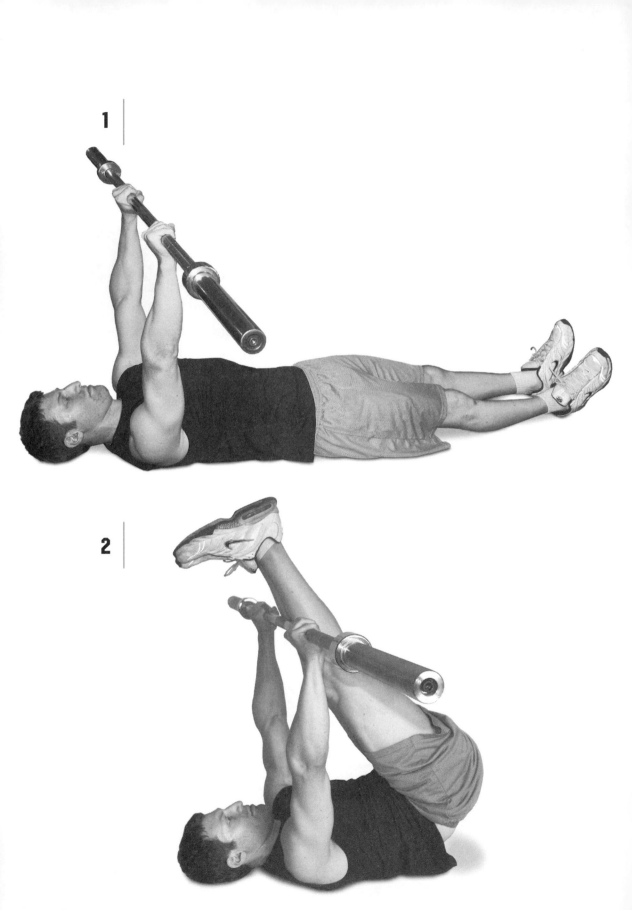

FLOOR WIPERS

Reps: 50

Description/Notes:

1 | Lie on the floor, face up. Hold the barbell out with straight arms at 90 degrees to your body in line with your chest.

2 | Lift up your legs, keeping them together and straight, so they touch the bar. Return them to the floor under control.

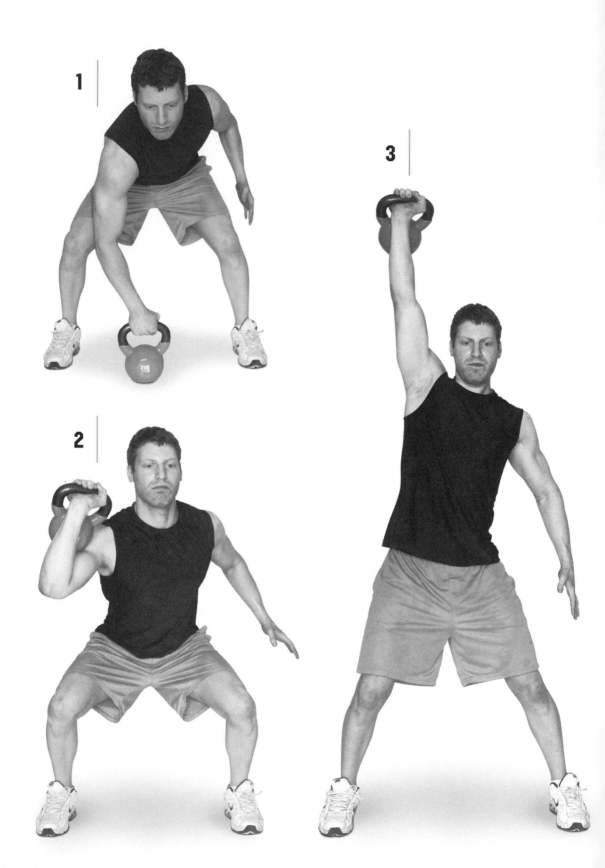

SINGLE-HAND KETTLEBELL CLEAN AND PRESS

Reps: 50 (25 each arm)

Description/Notes:

1	Position the kettlebell between your legs, back straight, knees bent.
2	Clean the kettlebell in one dynamic motion, and then press it above your head. Repeat 25 times for each arm.

To perform a kettlebell clean, pull the kettlebell up explosively, and when it reaches your mid thighs, shrug it up while simultaneously dropping yourself beneath it and performing what is effectively a reverse curl.

For a video of this exercise, visit:

www.youtube.com/watch?v=-T3FH3VNILo

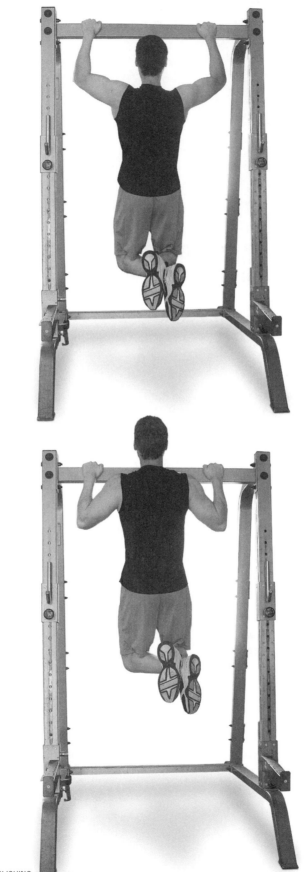

1

2

OVERHAND PULL-UPS

Reps: 25

Description/Notes:

1 | Find a pull-up bar high enough so your feet don't touch the floor. Assume an overhand grip on the bar.

2 | Pull up your body so your chin is above the bar then return under control until your arms are fully extended.

The "1 Rep Max" Test

The "1 Rep Max" test is a pure test of strength. The basic idea is to work out the maximum weight you can lift "once" for each of the ten exercises. You can record this weight for each exercise and use it to measure whether your strength has increased or decreased in certain muscle groups. As with the other two tests in this book, you should perform the "1 Rep Max" test at regular intervals during your training cycle, perhaps once every month. This way you can accurately gauge whether you are getting stronger.

Equipment Required

Various gym machines.

Instructions

Option 1:

Find the maximum weight you can lift for 1 repetition of each exercise. Note for First Timers: The first time you do this test it is really a process of finding out your limit. Start with a conservative estimate of what you think you can lift and try it out. If it is too light, increase the weight and try again until you reach your limit. Try to find your 1 repetition limit within 4 attempts; otherwise, it will not be a true reflection of your "1 Rep Max" limit.

Option 2:

If you are concerned that trying to lift as much weight as you can for 1 repetition may cause you to injure yourself, you can estimate the maximum weight you can lift by using a "1 Rep Max" Calculator. You insert a weight load and reps, and the calculator estimates your "1 Rep Max." Note: The fewer the reps entered into the calculator, the more accurate its results will be. **www.SportsWorkout.com/calculator**.

LEG PRESS

LEG EXTENSION

LEG CURL

DEAD LIFT

POSTERIOR DELTOID FLY

SEATED ROW

SHOULDER PRESS

LAT PULL-DOWN

BENCH PRESS

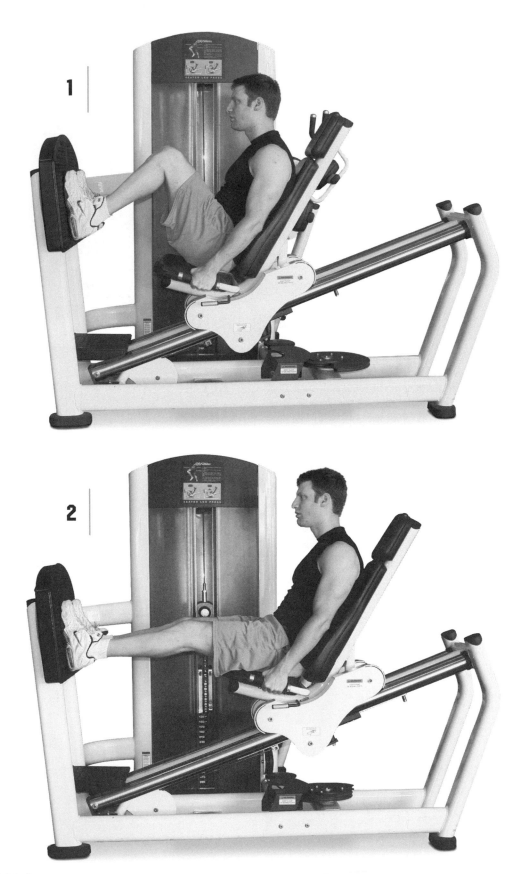

LEG PRESS

Reps: 1 (or more if necessary)

Description/Notes:

| 1 | Adjust seat position to suit your size. Take the weight off the rack, then slowly bring your knees down toward your chest. |
| 2 | Then push back up ensuring full range of motion. Do not lock out your knees, and do not put your hands on your knees (that's cheating!). |

For a video of this exercise, visit:

www.youtube.com/watch?v=TnOw3sUMyx8

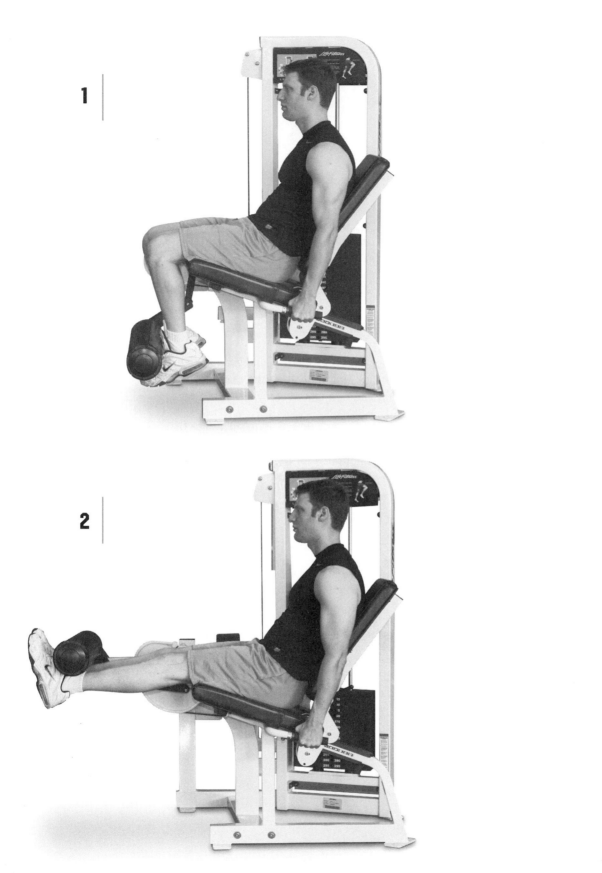

1

2

LEG EXTENSION

Reps: 1 (or more if necessary)

Description/Notes:

1	Adjust seat position to suit your size. Your knees should be in line with the pivot point of the machine.
2	Bring your legs up slowly in one continuous motion until they are straight, feet pointing upwards. Slowly return to the start position.

For a video of this exercise, visit:

www.youtube.com/watch?v=zCnMo2rhEo8

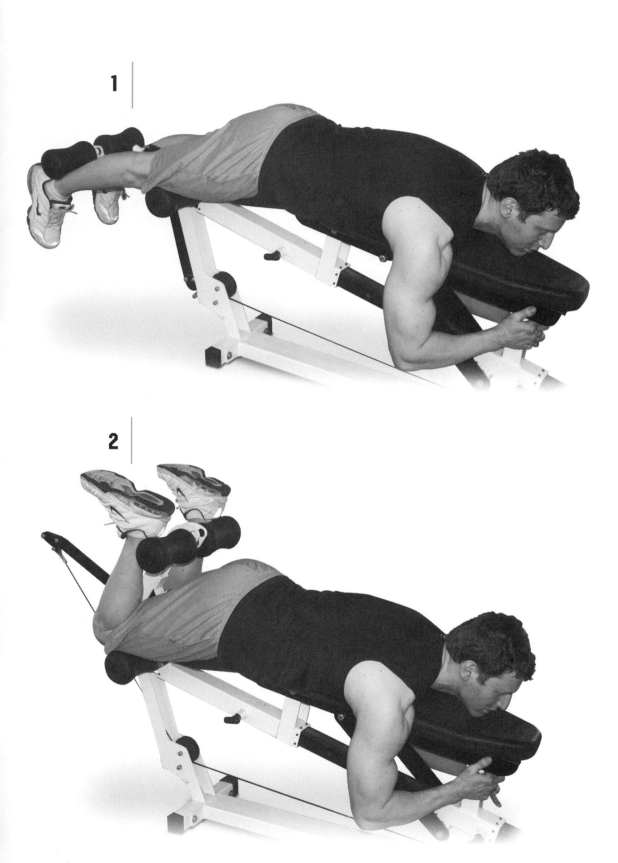

LEG CURL

Reps: 1 (or more if necessary)

Description/Notes:

1   Adjust seat position to suit your size. This can be done using a machine in the sitting or prone (lie face down) position. Here we will assume you are in the prone position. Lie down with your knees in line with the pivot point of the machine.

2   Bend your knees so your feet move up behind you until your legs are bent 90 degrees. Slowly return to the start position.

For a video of this exercise, visit:

www.youtube.com/watch?v=lmrIPrsH3iU

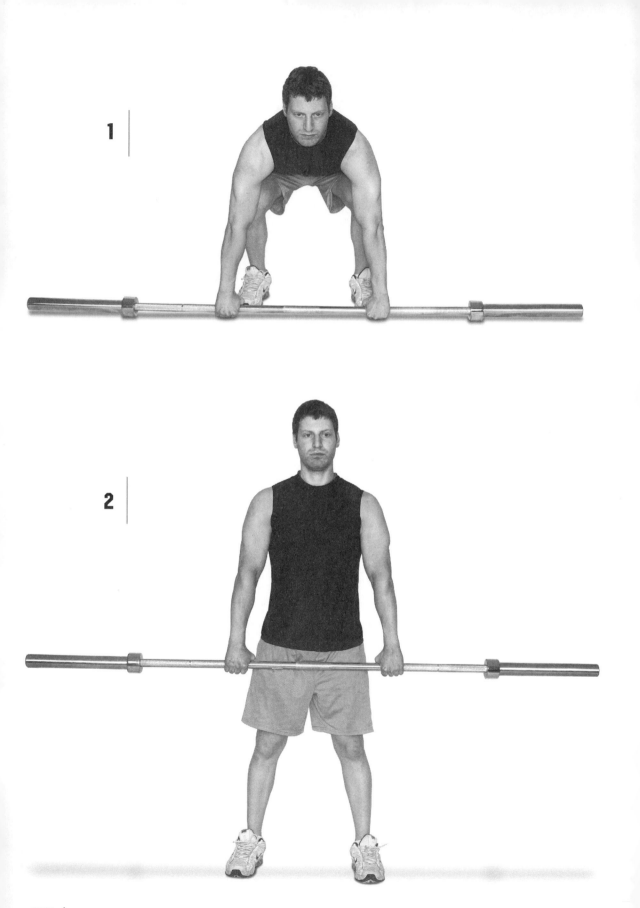

DEAD LIFT

Reps: 1 (or more if necessary)

Description/Notes:

1	Keeping your back straight, bend your knees and grip the barbell with both hands.
2	Lift the bar from the floor by straightening your knees until you are standing fully upright. Your back should remain straight throughout. Return the bar to the floor under control.

Technique is very important with this exercise to avoid injury.

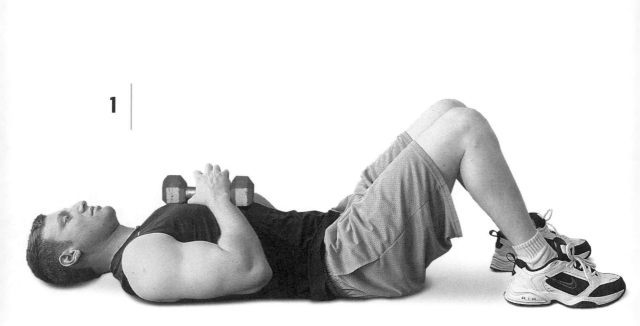

1

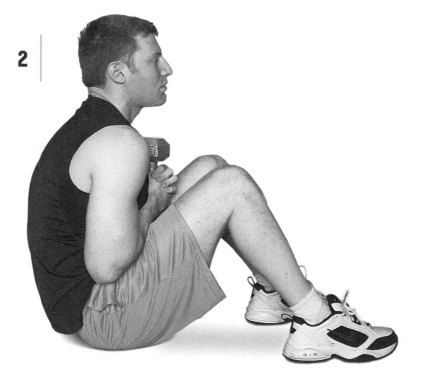

2

SIT-UP (USING DUMBBELL)

Reps: 1 (or more if necessary)

Description/Notes:

1 | Lie face up on the floor with your knees bent.

2 | Hold the dumbbell close to your chest, and then move your chest all the way up to your knees.

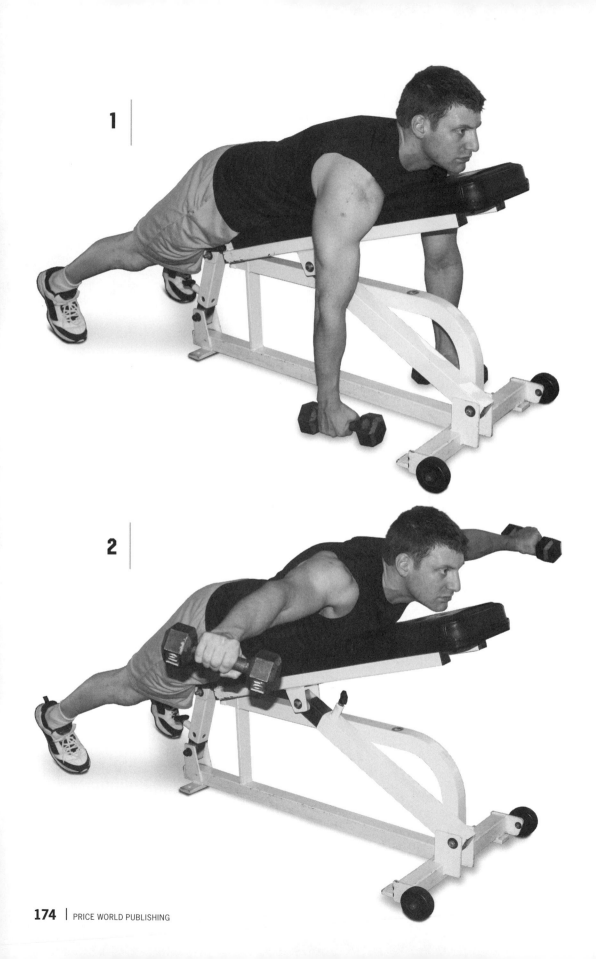

POSTERIOR DELTOID FLY

Reps: 1 (or more if necessary)

Description/Notes:

1 | Lie on an inclined bench in the prone position with your arms hanging of the bench.

2 | Extend your arms backward into a crucifix position. Exhale on the way back and inhale on the way in.

For a video of this exercise, visit:

www.youtube.com/watch?v=XCl8CfW_sxw

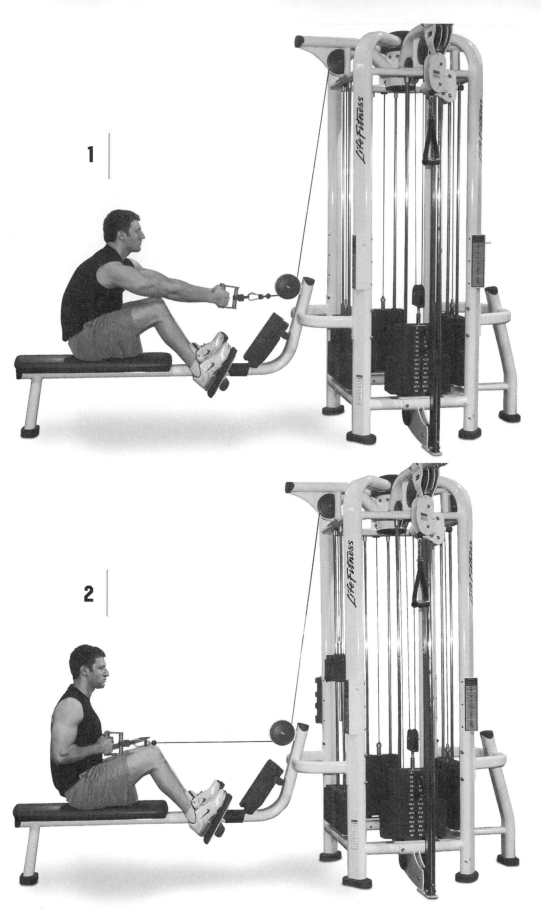

SEATED ROW

Reps: 1 (or more if necessary)

Description/Notes:

1 Adjust seat position to suit your size.
Grip the handles with your chest up and
shoulders down.

2 Pull the handles back toward your chest
ensuring full range of motion.
Slowly return to the start position.

For a video of this exercise, visit:

www.youtube.com/watch?v=Iz4F6jCyLc8

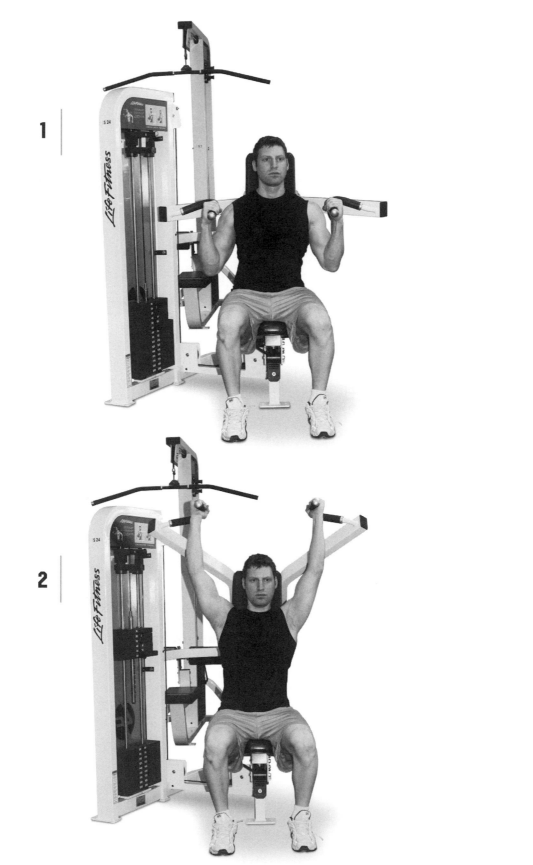

SHOULDER PRESS

Reps: 1 (or more if necessary)

Description/Notes:

1 This exercise can be done with a machine or free weights (dumbbells). Sit down, keep back straight. Hold the weight at your shoulders with your palms facing the ceiling.

2 Extend your arms, but do not lock out your elbows. Slowly return to the start position.

For a video of this exercise, visit:

www.youtube.com/watch?v=FpWrzp9Mnyg

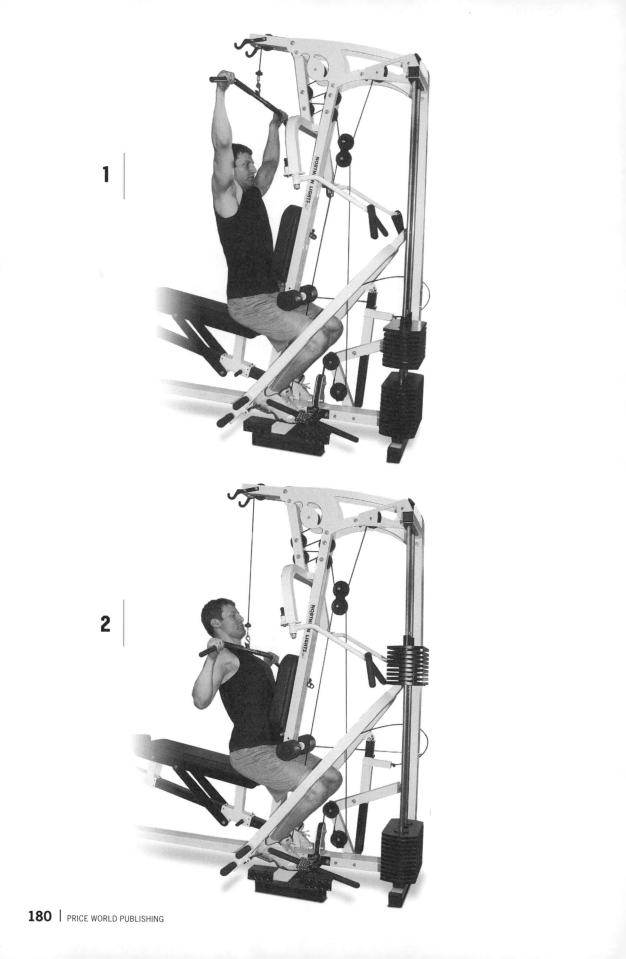

1

2

LAT PULL-DOWN

Reps: 1 (or more if necessary)

Description/Notes:

1	Adjust seat position to suit your size. Sit down so that your feet are flat on the ground and your back is straight.
2	Grip the bar above your head with a wide grip. Pull the bar down to your upper chest and slowly return to the start position.

For a video of this exercise, visit:

www.youtube.com/watch?v=UMC48BO-GQE

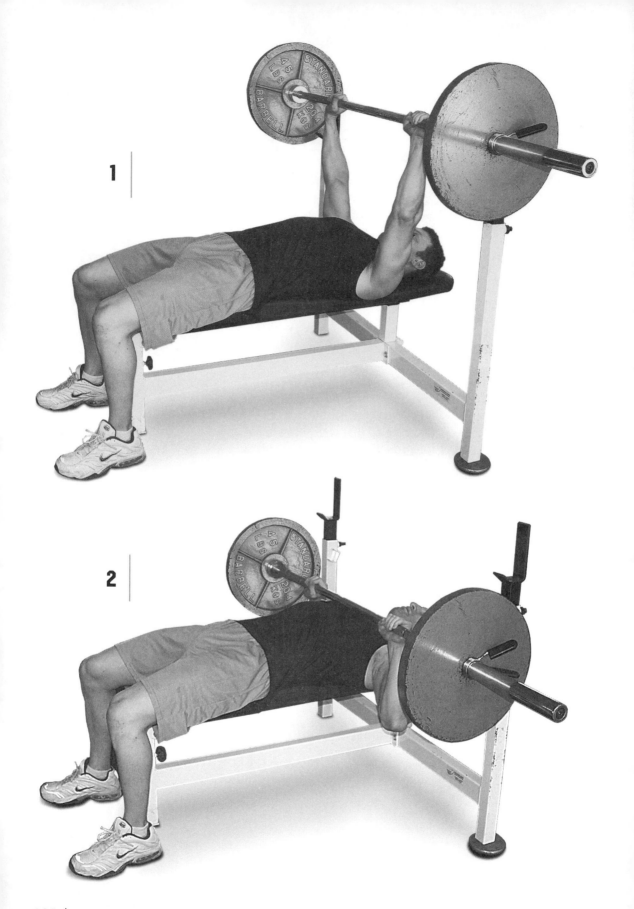

BENCH PRESS

Reps: 1 (or more if necessary)

Description/Notes:

1 | This exercise can be done with a chest press machine or a barbell. Lie down and grip the bar/handles. Keep your elbows in line with your shoulders.

2 | Extend your arms, but do not lock out your elbows. Slowly return to the start position.

For a video of this exercise, visit:

www.youtube.com/watch?v=tMOIT5vbFec

Training Logbook

Why bother keeping a logbook of your training? There are many reasons but probably the most important is that it lets you properly analyze the progress you are making toward your goals.

Without keeping track of key indicators like weight and heart rate, you will only be able to guess how much your fitness has improved.

Analyzing your diet is also important. Quite often you lose track of the snacks or small meals you consume. Only by writing it all down will you be able to see where you are going wrong, and then there shouldn't be any surprises when you step on the scales.

We recommend you start keeping a simply diary of your training and diet using the logbook pages we have provided for you online. You can print an unlimited supply of these pages by visiting **www.sportsworkout.com/hardcore**.

Each day the logbook is split into three separate areas.

In the first part, record your weight and resting heart rate. Resting heart rate means your heart rate during rest. This is best taken as soon as you get up in the morning.

The second part of the template lets you record the exercise you did, if any. Also you should record some key metrics: How long did you exercise for? What was your average heart rate during the exercise? Was there a result to record like a level for the bleep test?

If you cannot record your average heart rate during exercise (generally, you will only be able to do this with a heart rate monitor), then record your heart rate directly afterwards. Basically, you are just looking for an indication of how hard your training was.

The third part of the template allows you to comment on how intense you felt the exercise was (i.e., how hard you felt you worked), what you ate during the day, and any comments. Comments might include how you felt your training went or if you were sick or not quite on top form that day.

At the end of the week, there is a summary to fill in. This will allow you to make weekly comparisons. Did you train more than last week? Was your diet any better? Did your average resting heart rate decrease?

Finally, don't be disheartened if you don't see improvements over the first few weeks. Stick to it, put in the hard work, and you will reach your goals, given time.

HARDCORE CIRCUIT TRAINING FOR MEN | Body Weight Workout

DAY: **DATE:**   **BODY WT:**   **TOTAL TIME:**

RESTING H.R.:   **AVG H.R.:**   **COMMENTS:**

NUTRITION:

EXERCISE	WEIGHT & REPS	SET 1	SET 2	SET 3	SET 4
DYNAMIC "CLAP" PUSH-UPS	WEIGHT LOAD				
	PRESCRIBED REPS				
	COMPLETED REPS				
SINGLE ARM PUSH-UPS	WEIGHT LOAD				
	PRESCRIBED REPS				
	COMPLETED REPS				
"V" CRUNCH SIT-UPS	WEIGHT LOAD				
	PRESCRIBED REPS				
	COMPLETED REPS				
SIT-UPS	WEIGHT LOAD				
	PRESCRIBED REPS				
	COMPLETED REPS				
BACK EXTENSIONS	WEIGHT LOAD				
	PRESCRIBED REPS				
	COMPLETED REPS				
SINGLE-LEG "PISTOL" SQUATS	WEIGHT LOAD				
	PRESCRIBED REPS				
	COMPLETED REPS				
BURPEES WITH A JUMPING JACK	WEIGHT LOAD				
	PRESCRIBED REPS				
	COMPLETED REPS				

WEEKLY SUMMARY	TOTAL TRAINING TIME:	
Increases/decreases From Previous Week:	Nutrition Summary:	Training Notes:

Printable training logs can be found at www.sportsworkout.com/hardcore

Conclusion

This book is for guys who enjoy the challenge of hardcore physical training, but find it hard to fit exercise around their busy professional lives. We tell you everything you need to know about staying in peak physical condition while maintaining a healthy work/life balance. No nonsense, no fads, no BS - just practical, easy to remember workouts that make exercise enjoyable and challenging. With this book, boring gym visits will be a thing of the past!

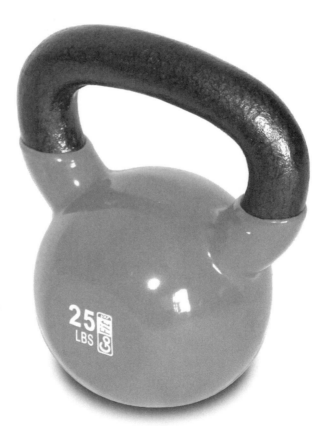

TRAINING NOTES

Index

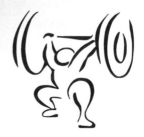